CURRENT REVIEWS IN OBSTETRICS AND GYNAECOLOGY

OBSTETRICS

Series Editor
Tom Lind MB BS DSc PhD MRCPath MRCOG
MRC Human Reproduction Group, Princess Mary Maternity Hospital, Newcastle upon Tyne

Volumes published
Obstetric Analgesia and Anaesthesia 2E *J. Selwyn Crawford*
Early Diagnosis of Fetal Defects *D. J. H. Brock*
Early Teenage Pregnancy *J. K. Russell*
Drug Prescribing in Pregnancy *B. Krauer, F. Krauer and F. Hytten*
Aspects of Care in Labour *J. M. Beazley and M. O. Lobb*
Spontaneous Abortion *H. J. Huisjes*
Coagulation Problems during Pregnancy *E. A. Letsky*

GYNAECOLOGY

Series Editors
Albert Singer DPhil PhD FRCOG
Whittington Hospital, London
Joe A. Jordan MD DObst FRCOG
Birmingham Maternity Hospital, Queen Elizabeth Medical Centre, Birmingham

Volumes published
Ovarian Malignancies *M. S. Piver*
Cancer of the Cervix *H. M. Shingleton and J. W. Orr*
Female Puberty and its Abnormalities *J. Dewhurst*
Infertility in the Male *A. M. Jequier*
Endometriosis *D. T. O'Connor*

Michael Brudenell
MBBS FRCS FRCOG
Consultant Obstetrician and Gynaecologist,
King's College Hospital, London

Marjorie Doddridge
MA MB BChir DRCOG
Associate Specialist, Diabetic Department,
King's College Hospital, London

Diabetic Pregnancy

Series Editor
TOM LIND

Churchill Livingstone 🕮

EDINBURGH LONDON MELBOURNE AND NEW YORK 1989

CHURCHILL LIVINGSTONE
Medical Division of Longman Group UK Limited

Distributed in the United States of America by Churchill
Livingstone Inc., 1560 Broadway, New York, N.Y. 10036,
and by associated companies, branches and representatives
throughout the world.

First published 1989

ISBN 0-443-02792-7

British Library Cataloguing in Publication Data

Brudenell, Michael
   Diabetic pregnancy
   1. Pregnant women. Diabetes.
   I. Title.   II. Doddridge, Marjorie C.
   III. Series
   618.3

Library of Congress Cataloging in Publication Data

Brudenell, Michael.
      Diabetic pregnancy/Michael Brudenell, Marjorie C. Doddridge.
      p.   cm. — (Current reviews in obstetrics and gynaecology,
   ISSN 0264-5610)
      Includes index.
      1. Diabetes in pregnancy.   I. Doddridge, Marjorie C.   II. Title.
   III. Series.
      [DNLM: 1. Pregnancy in Diabetes.   W1 CU8093M / WQ 248 B888d]
   RG580.D5B78 1989
   618.3 — dc19
   DNLM/DLC
   for Library of Congress   88-28548

Produced by Longman Singapore Publishers (Pte) Ltd.
Printed in Singapore

Preface

Before the advent of insulin very few diabetic women conceived and when they did the results were often disastrous for both mother and baby. In 1908 Offergeld could find only 57 cases of pregnancy complicated by maternal diabetes and in this series the perinatal mortality was 40% and maternal mortality 40%, the mothers dying in diabetic coma as a direct result of the pregnancy. Even as late as 1922 Joslin, an early pioneer in the treatment of diabetic pregnancy, could describe only 108 cases of diabetic pregnancy with a perinatal mortality rate of 44%.

Insulin was first isolated from the dog pancreas in 1921 by Banting, Best & McLeod, although the connection between the pancreas and spontaneous diabetes had been placed on a firm experimental basis by Meering & Minkowski 32 years previously in 1889. The first paper on the treatment of diabetes in man with insulin was published in 1922 by Banting & Best. In May 1923 Dr G Harrison, the biochemist at King's College Hospital, London, received a small supply of insulin from Canada and almost his first patient was Dr R D Lawrence, a King's doctor who had himself developed diabetes. Lawrence had to be hastily summoned back from Florence where he had gone as he supposed, to die in a rather more pleasant climate than that which prevailed in London. Successfully treated, Lawrence quickly established a diabetic clinic at King's and spent most of the rest of his long life working there treating diabetic patients. Once insulin was available maternal mortality in diabetic pregnancy fell sharply, but perinatal mortality remained high and was still in the region of 40% by the 1940s. Since that time, however, perinatal mortality has fallen steadily, with increasingly good control of the maternal diabetes and a better understanding of

v

the problems of the fetus. Of those who have contributed to the field of diabetic pregnancy, Priscilla White of Boston, Massachussetts (Joslin Clinic and Boston Hospital) is perhaps the most well known and has written extensively on the subject. In Europe the Rigs Hospitalet in Copenhagen has, for many years, been the main centre for diabetic pregnancy for the whole of Denmark and here many important contributions to the problem have been made, notably by Jorgen Pedersen & Mølsted-Pedersen. Bengt Persson in Sweden completes the notable Scandinavian trio who have done so much to increase understanding of the complexities of the subject. In the United States many workers have followed in the footsteps of Priscilla White: O'Sullivan's work on gestational diabetes, Freinkel's work on carbohydrate metabolism in pregnancy and latterly the work of Gabbe, Mestman & Jovanovic have maintained the North American tradition of expertise in the field. In Australia, Beischer and in South Africa Jackson & Coetzee have studied all aspects of diabetic pregnancy. At King's College Hospital, the early work of Lawrence in all aspects of diabetes, including diabetic pregnancy, was followed with a more detailed study by Dr Wilfred Oakley and Sir John Peel, who demonstrated the importance of a combined approach between diabetic physician and obstetrician in the management of diabetic pregnancy. This approach has been continued by the authors and Dr David Pyke and Dr Peter Watkins and the substance of this book is based upon the King's experience during the years 1971–85. Elsewhere in the British Isles, Beard at St Mary's Hospital, London, Gilmer at Oxford, Malins & Soler in Birmingham, Stowers and Sutherland in Aberdeen, Lind, Hytten & Alberti in Newcastle, Drury in Dublin as well as many others have made important contributions to the understanding and management of the problems encountered when a diabetic woman embarks on pregnancy. The worldwide interest in this unique situation in which the maternal disease affects and is affected by pregnancy justifies the large and continuing literature on the subject. This book attempts to look at the problem as it is seen at the present time and reports on the experience and current management policy in the diabetic pregnancy unit at King's College Hospital.

London, 1989

M.B.
M.D.

Contents

What is diabetes mellitus?

Diabetes mellitus is a clinical syndrome characterized by hyper-glycaemia due to a deficiency or diminished effectiveness of insulin. The metabolic disturbances affect the metabolism of carbohydrate, protein, fat, water and electrolytes. The deranged metabolism depends on the loss of insulin activity in the body and leads eventually, in many cases, to cellular damage, especially to vascular endothelial cells in the eye, kidney and nervous system. Diabetes mellitus is not a single disease but a group of diseases. The classification of diabetes mellitus suggested by the American National Diabetes Data Group in 1979 is generally accepted by the WHO (1980) (Table 1.1). The three main clinical types of interest to the obstetrician are insulin-dependent diabetes (IDD

Table 1.1 Classification of diabetes mellitus and other types of glucose intolerance (National Diabetes Data Group 1979)

Diabetes mellitus*	Insulin-dependent (IDD) or type 1 Non-insulin-dependent (NIDD) or type 2 Secondary diabetes with obesity without obesity
Diabetes with reduced glucose tolerance	
Gestational diabetes	
Prior abnormal glucose tolerance[†]	
Potentially abnormal glucose tolerance[†]	

* Based on fasting hyperglycaemia or an abnormal GTT.
[†] May be part of the natural history of diabetes. No alteration in carbohydrate metabolism.

or type I), non-insulin-dependent (NIDD or type II) and gestational diabetes. Potential diabetes is also of some relevance to obstetric practice but perhaps less important than was previously thought.

Non-Insulin-Dependent Diabetes (NIDD)

The majority of all diabetics are non-insulin dependent but NIDD is less common in the childbearing age group than in older women. There is an association between obesity and NIDD, which is more common in fat than in thin women. Obesity is associated with insulin insensitivity, and glucose tolerance improves with weight loss. However, most obese women are not diabetic and many NIDD patients are not obese, so the exact role of obesity in the pathogenesis of NIDD is uncertain. There is an hereditary element in NIDD; 25% of NIDD patients have a first degree family history of the disease and nearly all identical twins with NIDD have a similarly affected co-twin. Certain racial groups have a tendency to NIDD, especially those of Indian origin. In southern Africa NIDD is up to 20 times more common in Indians than in Africans (Mokgokong 1978). The decreased insulin response to a glucose challenge shown by many NIDD patients indicates a β cell deficiency. Insulin interacts with glycoprotein receptors on the cell surface. A combination of the hormone and its receptor is the first step in its action, resulting in the major action of insulin, which is to increase the transport of glucose across the membranes of insulin sensitive tissues especially liver, muscle and fat. NIDD patients, whether obese or not, have decreased numbers of insulin receptors and as a result have a decreased sensitivity and deficient response to insulin. The deterioration of glucose tolerance with age is probably due to similar receptor changes; insulin secretion does not lessen with age but sensitivity does. The NIDD woman has few symptoms and is not prone to ketosis but in pregnancy the management needs to be just as careful as for IDD patients if perinatal losses are to be avoided.

Insulin-Dependent Diabetes (IDD)

This type of diabetes occurs most often in young adults; the prevalence rate varies but is about 0.2% in whites under the age of 30. It is unusual in the newborn but the incidence rises with increasing age to reach a peak at 11–14 years. Thereafter, the incidence declines slowly to a plateau of about 8 per 100 000 (Lernmark 1985). Shortly after the diagnosis of IDD has been made, inflammatory cells are found infiltrating and surrounding the islets of Langerhans, so-called insulitis. There is a marked decrease in the number of β cells. A number of factors are involved in the aetiology of IDD; genetic determinants involve certain histocompatibility antigens (HLA) on chromosome 6 (Cudworth & Woodrow 1976), especially HLA-DR3 and DR4 which are associated with an increased incidence of IDD. Given that these genetic markers indicate an increased susceptibility to diabetes for the individuals concerned there are a number of possible initiators of the disease, including environmental factors and viruses such as the Coxsackie B4 and Rubella as well as chemicals such as streptozotocin and certain rodenticides.

An immune response in IDD patients is expressed by the presence of islet cell cytoplasmic antibodies (ICA) and islet cell surface antibodies (ICSA). These antibodies are found in the majority of IDD patients at the time of diagnosis and in the case of ICA this may be present 2–7 years before the condition is diagnosed. (The value of a positive ICA test for the prediction of IDD will depend on accurate and reproducible ICA tests becoming generally available. When and if they do so, screening of susceptible women, e.g. those with a positive family history, might be of considerable value to the obstetrician). Thus IDD patients have a cellular and humoral autoimmunity to pancreatic β cells.

The current hypothesis as to the cause of the IDD is that the combination of specific antigen molecules coded by the HLA genes DR, DQ and DP with an invading antigen, virus, bacterium or chemical triggers the formation of effector cells such as B lymphocytes and cytotoxic T lymphocytes which cross-react with the islet β cells. The loss of sufficient numbers of islet β cells precipitates IDD (Lernmark 1985). The extent to which residual β cells function exists in the pregnant IDD has been investigated by Pirthiaho et al (1986), who found increased serum C peptide immunoreactivity (CPR) in 23 IDD women throughout pregnancy. CPR values generally increased at 23–33 weeks onwards. When the women were divided into two groups on the basis of residual β cell function as shown by CPR levels, the glycaemic control was better in the group with the greatest residual β cell function. The authors suggest that pregnancy enhances residual β cell function, which may be of clinical importance in ensuring good glycaemic control.

Diagnosis of diabetes mellitus (Table 1.2)

In a patient with symptoms the essentially arbitrary diagnosis of diabetes mellitus is established by a raised fasting blood glucose level in venous plasma of 8 mmol/l or more or 11 mmol/l or more after food. A fasting level of less than 6 mmol/l usually excludes the diagnosis of diabetes. When the fasting level is between 6 and 8 mmol/l a glucose tolerance test (GTT) should be performed. Although there are variations in oral GTTs and an extensive literature on intravenous GTTs the 75 g oral GTT, as advocated by the WHO (1980), is likely to become the most widely used in the future and has the virtue of simplicity in interpretation. A standard load of 75 g glucose in 250 ml water is given after an overnight fast following 3 days of adequate carbohydrate intake (greater than 250 g/day). Blood samples are taken before and at 1 and 2 hours after the load. The test distinguishes between normal diabetes mellitus and impaired glucose tolerance (IGT). The latter has particular relevance in pregnancy, for some women with IGT in early pregnancy may progress to diabetes in late pregnancy.

Table 1.2 Diagnostic glucose concentrations

Diagnosis	Venous blood in mmol/l	Capillary whole blood in mmol/l	Venous plasma in mmol/l
Diabetes mellitus*			
Fasting	≥ 7.0	≥ 7.0	≥ 8.0
2 hour blood glucose	≥10.0	≥11.0	≥11.0
Impaired glucose tolerance			
Fasting	< 7.0	< 7.0	< 8.0
2 hour blood glucose	≥ 7.0–<10.0	≥ 8.0–<11.0	≥ 8.0–<11.0

* In the absence of diabetic symptoms an abnormal 1 hour level is required in addition to the 2 hour figure to confirm the diagnosis of diabetes mellitus (WHO 1980).

Gestational diabetes (GDM) and impaired glucose tolerance (IGT) in pregnancy

Traditionally, gestational diabetes was a term applied to women who became diabetic during pregnancy and reverted to normal thereafter. Recently, the term has been applied to women who become diabetic in pregnancy regardless of whether or not they return to normal once the pregnancy is over. Many women who develop diabetes in pregnancy do revert to normal post partum but some do not; the two groups may thus differ in epidemiological terms, representing two distinct populations. For this reason some authors (Essex & Pyke 1978) preferred to use the term 'diabetes diagnosed in pregnancy'. From the obstetrician's point of view the distinction between the two groups is probably academic for if a woman becomes truly diabetic in pregnancy, i.e. gestational diabetic in modern parlance, the pregnancy is at once at risk, regardless of the eventual post-partum maternal status, and there is, at present, no clear evidence that the course of the pregnancy is affected by whether or not the patient remains diabetic post partum or reverts to normal. The definition of diabetes proposed by the WHO and outlined earlier in this chapter is acceptable to most diabetic physicians and obstetricians, as is the proposal for an intermediate group of individuals whose carbohydrate metabolism does not constitute gestational diabetes but is not entirely normal.

'Impaired glucose tolerance' has the merit of being factual and of identifying a group of women who may progress to gestational diabetes as the pregnancy advances or who may remain with impairment of carbohydrate metabolism until the end of the pregnancy, reverting to normal thereafter. The significance of IGT to the obstetrician has been much debated, but providing it remains within the WHO criteria laid down it seems it is unusual for it to have any adverse effect on the clinical course of the pregnancy. This view is, however, at variance with a recent report by Tallarigo et al (1986), who studied the frequency of maternal complications (toxaemia, caesarean section) and fetal problems (macrosomia, congenital abnormality and perinatal mortality) in relation to glucose tolerance in the third trimester of pregnancy in 249 women. The women were non-diabetic by normal testing but were divided into three categories according to their 2-hour glucose level response to a 100 g glucose load. The incidence of both maternal and fetal complications, though not perinatal mortality or prematurity, increased as the 2-hour figure rose, indicating that even limited degrees of maternal hyperglycaemia may influence pregnancy outcome. This paper also illustrates the problem of definition: had the authors been using a WHO recommended 75 g glucose load and obtained similar 2-hour levels, some at least of their patients would have come into the IGT category. For the present, it would seem prudent to regard any abnormality of carbohydrate metabolism with suspicion although, except for fetal macrosomia, serious adverse effects are unlikely to arise, certainly if the glucose tolerance of the pregnant woman in the third trimester is normal by WHO standards and probably for the majority of those IGT women whose glucose tolerance does not deteriorate as pregnancy advances.

Practical considerations are likely to determine how individual obstetricians screen for and manage gestational diabetes and impaired glucose tolerance. The latter condition will only be detected if some form of blood glucose measurement is employed as a screening method, so the obstetrician who relies on urine testing and clinical diagnosis alone is not going to be bothered by it, although he will certainly be faced with a number of true gestational diabetics. When screening tests are employed impaired glucose tolerance will be detected in about 3% or less of most clinic populations. If the impairment remains unchanged throughout the remainder of the pregnancy (and the patient must have regular fasting blood glucose estimations to confirm this) as indicated above, no treatment is necessary, since there is little or no increased fetal risk (Hadden 1980). The true gestational diabetic is a different proposition: her risks are similar to those of the established diabetics and she must be treated with or without insulin depending on the severity of the diabetes and managed in the combined diabetic antenatal clinic if fetal loss is to be avoided.

The fetal risk is underlined by the King's experience. In the early series 1951–70 the perinatal mortality in gestational diabetes (16.6%) was almost the same as for established diabetics (15.5%). Latterly, with the realisation that gestational diabetes posed a similar threat to the fetus, the perinatal mortality for gestational diabetes in 1971–80 had fallen to 1.5%, half that for established diabetics in the same period (3.3%). In the period 1981–85 there were no perinatal deaths in gestational diabetics (Table 1.3). The effect of diabetic complications in established

Table 1.3 Perinatal mortality in gestational and established diabetes at King's College Hospital

	Established diabetics	Gestational diabetics
1951–70	15.5%	16.6%
1971–80	3.3%	1.5%
1981–85	1.2%	0.0%

diabetics on perinatal mortality is discussed in Chapter 3.

The long-term follow-up of women with gestational diabetes has been studied by Grant et al (1986), who retested 447 women who had gestational diabetes at intervals from 1 to 12 years following diagnosis; 49 (11%) were found to be diabetic and 35 (7.8%) had IGT. Obesity, an impaired GTT in the puerperium and recurrence of gestational diabetes in a subsequent pregnancy were significant factors in the later development of diabetes or IGT. Farrell et al (1986) found a higher frequency of abnormal glucose tolerance in gestational diabetics tested up to 12 months after delivery: 14 of the 42 (33.3%) GDM patients had an abnormal GTT, 10 (26%) being frankly diabetic.

Potential abnormality of glucose tolerance

Certain groups of women are more likely to develop diabetes mellitus at some time during their lifetime than normal, and are labelled potential diabetics. From the obstetrician's point of view the risk that these individuals will develop gestational diabetes or impaired glucose tolerance in pregnancy is low, but the risk factors remain useful criteria in clinical screening where routine screening of the whole antenatal population is not carried out. The risk factors that are important to the obstetrician are detailed below.

Family history

As noted above, genetic factors play a part in the development of diabetes, although the exact mode of inheritance is not established. Approximately 1% of all offspring of an IDD parent may be expected to develop the disease themselves in the first 30 years of life, an incidence of between 5 and 10 times greater than that of a child with non-diabetic parents. A history of IDD in the father is of greater predictive value than in the mother, and even greater when a sibling is diabetic. Family history in grandparents is less significant. If both parents are diabetic the incidence of diabetes in the offspring rises, depending upon the age at which the parents became diabetic. The greatest risk of the offspring developing diabetes occurs when one or both parents develop the disease before the age of 40. Even so, not more than 25% of their children will become diabetic and the figure is lower in children of parents with diabetes of late onset. The extent to which a positive family history makes an individual a potential diabetic will therefore vary with circumstances (Pyke 1968).

Previous heavy babies

The incidence of babies weighing 4.5 kg or more is about 5% of all births. Among the children of women who later develop diabetes the figure is much higher, varying in different reports from 4% to 31% (Pyke 1962). A tendency to bear heavy babies may precede the development of clinical diabetes by many years. There is no clear-cut evidence to support the idea that the proportion of heavy babies increases as the time of diagnosis draws near, suggesting that genetic factors are more important than environmental factors, particularly maternal hyperglycaemia. Women who develop an abnormal glucose tolerance in pregnancy may produce a heavier than average baby but, if treated with diet or insulin, they may not (O'Sullivan, Gellis & Tenney 1966). Apart from the genetic and environmental influences exerted by the mother, the father might theoretically exert a genetic influence on the birthweight of his offspring. There is no convincing evidence that men who subsequently become diabetic father heavier babies than normal in their prediabetic phase or, indeed, once they become established diabetics.

Obesity

Women who are obese (weight exceeds 90 kg) have a greater tendency to become diabetic in later life than non-obese women. From the practical point of view the most important aspect is the probability that any one individual will develop diabetes or impaired glucose tolerance in the future. Unless this occurs during pregnancy, the condition is of academic interest only to the obstetrician. For the patient herself, the risk is of great importance but is one that is not easy to quantify because of the lack of controlled prospective studies. In a study reported by Pedersen (1977) women who had given birth to a baby weighing 4.5 kg or more 20 years previously with no family history had an incidence of diabetes of 17% if they were of normal weight and a 46% incidence if they were obese. Women who had given birth to a big baby who were both obese and had a positive family history had an incidence of diabetes of 84%. Thus the prognostic significance of having given birth to big babies was connected both with the family history and obesity. When the three features occur together, the risk of subsequent diabetes is high. For women who have big babies but who are not obese and do not have a family history, the risk of developing diabetes is probably not much greater than normal.

Classification of severity of diabetes in pregnancy

In general terms, the more severe the diabetes the greater the risk of maternal complications in pregnancy and perinatal mortality and morbidity. Severity in this context is measured by the presence of diabetic vascular complications and by the duration of the diabetes. Traditionally, the classification used is that of White (1965), but this now seems unnecessarily complicated. At King's College Hospital, since 1971, classification based on the severity of vascular complications instead of the White classification has been used. There are three groups:

Group 1: Diabetes diagnosed during pregnancy (synonymous with gestational diabetes in most modern publications);
Group 2: Established diabetes with six or less microaneurysms seen on opthalmoscopy;
Group 3: Established diabetes with more than six microaneurysms or proliferative retinopathy and/or nephropathy.

This simple classification indicates the distribution of diabetic pregnancies by 'severity' of maternal disease in a given population and the effect which 'severity' has on clinical outcome,

Diabetic pregnancy

Table 1.4 Classification of diabetic mothers 1981–85

	IDD	NIDD	TOTAL
GROUP I Gestational	1	32	33 17%
GROUP II Established	116	17	133 69%
GROUP III Established with complications	27	0	27 14%
TOTAL	144 75%	49 25%	193

particularly perinatal mortality. The distribution of diabetic mothers, insulin dependent and non-insulin dependent, at King's College Hospital in 1981–85 is shown in Table 1.4. No NIDD patient came into the group 3 category, indicating the rarity with which these patients develop vascular complications.

REFERENCES

Cudworth A G, Woodrow J C 1976 Genetic susceptibility in diabetes mellitus: analysis of the HLA association. British Medical Journal 2: 1333–1336

Essex N, Pyke D A 1978 Management of maternal diabetes in pregnancy. Carbohydrate metabolism in pregnancy and the newborn. Springer–Verlag, Berlin, pp 357–368

Farrell J, Forest J M, Storey G N, Yue D K, Shearman R P, Turte J R 1986 Gestational diabetes, infant malformations and subsequent maternal glucose tolerance. Australian and New Zealand Journal of Obstetrics and Gynaecology 26 (1): 11–16

Grant P T, Oats J N, Beischer N H 1986 The long term follow up of women with gestational diabetes. Australian and New Zealand Journal of Obstetrics and Gynaecology 26 (1): 17–22

Hadden D R 1980 Screening for abnormalities of carbohydrate metabolism in pregnancy. The Belfast experience. Diabetes Care 3: 440–446

Lernmark A 1985 Causes of insulin dependent diabetes. Medicine International 13: 535–538

Mokgokong E D 1978 Some clinical and biochemical features of pregnant African diabetics and comparison of their features with those of pregnant Indian diabetics. MD thesis. University of Natal, Durban

National Diabetes Data Group 1979 Classification and diagnosis of diabetes mellitus and other categories of glucose intolerance. Diabetes 28: 1039–1057

O'Sullivan J B, Gellis S S, Tenney B O 1966 The potential diabetic and her treatment in pregnancy. Diabetes 15: 466

Pedersen J 1977 The pregnant diabetic and her newborn, 2nd edn. Williams & Williams, Baltimore, p 52

Pirthiaho H I, Hartikaenen-Sorri A L, Kuila J M, Puuka R 1986 Residual cell function and glycaemic control in diabetic pregnancy. Hormone Metabolism Research 18, 4: 250–252

Pyke D A 1962 Disorders of carbohydrate metabolism. Pitman, London
Pyke D A 1968 In: Oakley W G, Pyke D A, Taylor K W (eds) Clinical diabetes. Blackwell, Oxford, p 220–221
Tallarigo L, Gianpreto O, Penno G et al 1986 Relation of glucose tolerance to complications in pregnancy in non-diabetic women. New England Journal of Medicine 315(16): 989–992
White P 1965 Pregnancy and diabetes: medical aspects. Medical Clinics. North America 49: 1015
WHO Expert Committee on Diabetes 1980 Second report. WHO Technical Report Series 646, Geneva

2

Carbohydrate and lipid metabolism in pregnancy

From a clinical standpoint, the central features of carbohydrate and lipid metabolism can be summarized in simple terms. When a woman becomes pregnant she needs more insulin to maintain normal carbohydrate metabolism. If she is unable to produce more insulin to meet the demand she may become diabetic, with the resultant changes in both her carbohydrate and lipid metabolisms—the latter being consequent on the former. The level of glucose in the woman's blood is a measure of her ability to respond to this challenge of pregnancy. The maternal blood glucose level is reflected in the fetal blood glucose level, since glucose crosses the placenta easily. The same is true of maternal and fetal levels of lipids. Insulin does not cross the placental barrier, so that excess production of insulin by mother or fetus remains with the producer. Finally, glycosuria is commoner in pregnant than in non-pregnant women, a factor of considerable importance in considering the detection and control of diabetes in pregnancy.

In order to have a better understanding of the changes simply described in the above paragraph, it is important to examine the mechanism by which carbohydrate and lipid metabolisms change in normal pregnancy.

Carbohydrate and lipid metabolism in normal pregnancy

Hormonal changes

Extensive hormone changes occur in pregnancy in order to maintain the metabolic state of the mother (Table 2.1). The ovary,

Table 2.1 Hormone changes in pregnancy which affect carbohydrate metabolism

Oestrogen Progesterone HPL(HCS) Free cortisol Prolactin }	Rise progressively
Insulin	Rises slowly to 32 weeks. Declines thereafter to near non-pregnant levels
Glucagon	Unchanged or slight rise

the fetal adrenal cortex, the placenta, the anterior pituitary, the maternal adrenal cortex, and the pancreas are all involved in bringing about these hormone changes, which have a profound effect on both carbohydrate and lipid metabolism. Of particular importance is the progressive rise in circulating oestrogen produced initially by the ovary up to the 9th week of intrauterine life and thereafter by the placenta. The fetal adrenal contributes dehydroepiandrosterone sulphate, the precursor steroid for oestrogen in the latter half of pregnancy. The majority of oestrogen formed by the placenta is in the form of free oestriol, which is conjugated in the liver to the more soluble glucuronides and sulphates, which are excreted in the urine (Telgedy et al 1962). Progesterone is produced throughout pregnancy by the corpus luteum but especially during the first 6 weeks. The trophoblast synthesizes progesterone from maternal cholesterol and is the main contributor to the steadily increasing level of plasma progesterone during pregnancy (Ryan, Meigs & Petro 1966). Human placental lactogen (HPL), also known as human chorionic somatomammotrophin (HCS), is the other important placental hormone affecting carbohydrate metabolism. Its level in the maternal blood increases gradually throughout pregnancy, reaching a peak at term. It has a short half-life (29 min), so that maternal blood concentrations fall to zero soon after the placenta is delivered (Tyson et al 1972). The anterior pituitary causes a rise in prolactin levels from the 9th week onwards in parallel with oestrogen levels, reaching a peak at term. Levels remain high after delivery if the woman breastfeeds, declining only after several months of lactation (Telgedy et al 1962). The adrenal cortex brings about a rise in the levels of free cortisol progressively throughout pregnancy (Gemzell 1953). In mid- and late pregnancy this is not due to increased secretion by the adrenal but to a reduction in metabolic clearance by the liver as a result of the high oestrogen levels (Burke & Roulet 1970).

Pregnancy is accompanied by a significant hypertrophy of the β-islet cells of the pancreas, probably as a result of increased oestrogen and progesterone levels (Hellman 1960, Aerts & Van Asshe 1975). Experimental work on rats has demonstrated an increase in size of β-cells and their secretion of insulin following administration of 17β-oestradiol or progesterone separately or in combination, indicating a direct effect upon the β-cells of the endocrine pancreas (Costrini & Kalkhoff 1971). Green & Taylor (1972) showed that β-cells are more sensitive to the stimulating effects of glucose in pregnancy, i.e. more insulin is put out for a given blood glucose concentration. This is presumably due to the raised level of other pregnancy hormones, including oestrogen, progesterone and HPL. If pregnant women consume more carbohydrate, and they often do, any extra glucose arriving at the β-cells would trigger increased β-cell activity quite apart from any direct stimulating effect of other hormones. Pregnancy has little or no effect on the α-cells. In human pregnancy the level of fasting insulin in the circulating blood rises slowly. Baird (1986), reporting on a longitudinal study involving 86 normal pregnant women whose 3-hour post-prandial levels of plasma glucose (PG) and plasma immunoreactive insulin (IRI) were measured serially at <12, 16, 33 weeks' gestation and 6 weeks post partum, found a progressive rise in the IRI : PG ratio to a peak at 32 weeks and a gradual decline thereafter to non-pregnant levels post partum. Glucagon levels, as might be expected are unchanged or show only a slight rise in pregnancy (Luyckx et al 1975, Kühl & Holst 1976).

Carbohydrate metabolism

Mainly as a result of the hormonal changes described above, carbohydrate metabolism in pregnancy undergoes characteristic changes (Table 2.2). Lind et al (1973) and Victor (1974) reported that the fasting level of glucose is slightly but significantly lower than normal from the tenth week onwards. Baird (1986), in the study mentioned above, found a small but significant rise in fasting blood glucose levels from 16 to 32 weeks and a fall thereafter, so that at term the glucose level was not significantly different from that found in matched non-pregnant controls. The

Table 2.2 Carbohydrate metabolism changes in pregnancy

Glucose	Fasting level initially low then rises slowly to 32 weeks: declines thereafter; peak levels higher
Intravenous glucose tolerance	Increased disappearance rate in early pregnancy; normal in late pregnancy
Insulin response to glucose	Unchanged in first and second trimester; increased in third trimester
Renal handling of glucose	Increased GFR; diminished tubular reabsorption hence increased glycosuria

peak levels of glucose after a carbohydrate load are higher than normal, especially after the 20th week (Lind, Billewicz & Brown 1973, Kühl C 1975). Nevertheless, in normal human pregnancy blood glucose levels are kept within a relatively narrow range which cannot be matched by the diabetic woman, no matter how well her diabetes is controlled.

The pattern of change in the response to an intravenous injection of glucose is interesting in that the rate of disappearance of glucose is increased in early pregnancy and returns to a normal level in late pregnancy (Pedersen 1977). The insulin response to oral or intravenous glucose is substantially increased during the third trimester of pregnancy (Bleicher, O'Sullivan & Freinkl 1964, Fischer P M et al 1974). In the second half of pregnancy, especially during the third trimester, there is an increase in insulin antagonism with a slight deterioration in glucose tolerance, and the hypoglycaemic effect of intravenous insulin is less (Burt 1956). Gestational diabetes is most commonly seen at this time and in the rare conditions of a pre-existing insulin-secreting adenoma in pregnancy, the episodes of hypoglycaemia are diminished (Hagin 1961). The mechanism of insulin resistance is unclear but normal pregnant women, gestational diabetics and insulin-dependent diabetics all exhibit the phenomenon (Kühl 1975, Baird 1986).

Gray, quoted by Baird (1986), using the euglycaemic insulin clamp technique to compare insulin action in insulin-treated diabetics during the third trimester and post partum, showed that the glucose disposal rate post partum was 60% greater in spite of a 30% lower mean peripheral free insulin concentration. The fetus disposes of a substantial proportion of glucose, independent of insulin action, so the degree of resistance to the peripheral action of insulin in the mother has probably been underestimated. There is no alteration in insulin receptor binding in erythrocytes or monocytes (Tsiblis et al 1980, Moore et al 1981, Pedersen et al 1981, Puavilai et al 1982). In the rat, Flint et al (1979) have shown that the number of insulin receptors on adipocytes in the rat is doubled but there is no information regarding insulin receptors on adipocytes, skeletal muscle cells or hepatocytes in man.

The impaired responsiveness to injected insulin has been interpreted as a post-receptor defect in insulin action (Kahn 1978), perhaps related to the rising level of HPL (HCS), although the rising level of cortisol as well as other pregnancy hormones may also play a part (Ursell, Brudenell & Chard 1973). The net increase in insulin action on carbohydrate metabolism in early human pregnancy conserves energy—'facilitated anabolism'—is reduced in later pregnancy so as to provide ample glucose to the fetus at a time when its growth is maximal and its peferential utilization of this substance reaches a peak (Metzger & Frankel 1975).

Feto-maternal blood glucose relationships

Glucose crosses the placental barrier by the process of facilitated diffusion, and the fetal blood glucose level closely follows the maternal level. The glucose transport mechanism protects the fetus from excessively high maternal levels, becoming saturated by maternal glucose levels of 10 mmol/l or more so that the fetal blood glucose level peaks at 8–9 mmol/l. This ensures that in normal pregnancy the fetal pancreas is not overstimulated by post-prandial peaks in the maternal blood glucose levels (Beard, Turner & Oakley 1971, Oakley, Beard & Turner 1972).

Renal handling of glucose

Glycosuria is common in pregnancy, starting within 6 weeks of the last menstrual period. The mean excretion rate of glucose per 24 hours is 76 mg in the pregnant woman. A minority of women secrete significantly larger amounts of glucose, up to 1 g or more in 24 hours in the last 4 weeks of pregnancy. There is a tendency for glycosuria to increase as pregnancy advances, but there is a great deal of diurnal and day-to-day variation in excretion rate.

There is no constant relationship in normal pregnancy between urinary and blood glucose levels. The reason for the increase in glucose excretion in pregnancy is complex, but it is mainly due to an increased glomerular filtration rate (GFR) and a diminished ability by the proximal, and perhaps also the distal renal tubules, to reabsorb glucose. There is almost certainly a hormonal basis for these changes, since they decline rapidly after delivery, as does glucose excretion. This does not, however, explain the intermittent nature of pregnancy glycosuria (Lind & Hytten 1972, Davison 1974, Davison & Hytten 1975).

Lipid metabolism

Every aspect of lipid metabolism is affected by pregnancy, particularly the free fatty acids, triglycerides, phospholipids and cholesterol.

Free fatty acid (FFA), triglycerides and glycerol

The plasma level of FFA falls from early to mid-pregnancy and thereafter shows a significant rise. The same is true of the plasma level of glycerol. This is in keeping with the accumulation of body fat that occurs during the first two trimesters of pregnancy (anabolic phase). In the last trimester increased catabolism occurs, causing raised FFA and glycerol levels which are then available as fuel to the maternal tissues to offset the increasing diversion to the rapidly growing fetus of glucose and amino acids. The increased level of FFA also leads to an increase in the transplacental passage to the fetus (Goldstein et al 1985). There is a temporary fall in both FFA and glycerol levels immediately post partum, followed by a rise during breastfeeding, presumably to allow a similar diversion of the ingested maternal nutrients for the synthesis of breast milk. Free fatty acid has a high energy yield and is especially important as a fuel for skeletal and cardiac muscle, sparing glucose and other non-lipids from utilization by these tissues. It also provides an important substrate to be converted in the liver to triglyceride and ketone bodies. In late pregnancy the plasma level of triglyceride is raised and there is a tendency to ketosis. Since some of the additional FFA crosses the placenta, the fetus also benefits from the additional substrate made available to its liver and for tissue lipogenesis. In this respect the glucose-saving property of FFA in maternal metabolism is mirrored in the fetus (Kalkhoff, Kissebah & Hak Joong 1979).

Cholesterol and phospholipid

As as with FFA, glycerol and triglycerides, the plasma levels of cholesterol and phospholipid are increased. The increase in the former accounts for the predisposition of the pregnant woman to gallstones, especially as there is a relative reduction in the excretion of bile acids (O'Sullivan, Walker & Bondar 1975). The significance of the change in cholesterol and phospholipid metabolism in pregnancy is not clear but, as with the other changes in fat and carbohydrate metabolism, it is mediated by hormonal changes and fits into the general pattern of an increase in storage of glycogen and fat in most maternal tissues during the first two trimesters of pregnancy. In the third trimester, the storage of nutrients levels off and more fuel is mobilized for the benefit of both mother and fetus (Kalkhoff, Kissebah & Hak Joon 1979).

Conclusion

The biphasic metabolic pattern of conservation of energy in maternal tissue in the first half of pregnancy, with the redirection of available energy for the benefit of the mother and especially the fetus in the second half, is mainly under the control of the placental steroids and is independent of maternal diet. This internal redistribution of substrate in the two halves of pregnancy under hormonal control is the main characteristic of the maternal metabolic adaptation to pregnancy. The precise mechanisms underlying these adjustments have still to be defined (Baird 1986).

REFERENCES

Aerts L, Van Asshe F A 1975 Ultrastructural changes of the endocrine pancreas in pregnant rats. Diabetologia 11: 285–289

Baird J D 1986 Some aspects of metabolism and hormonal adaptation to pregnancy. Acta Endocrinologica Suppl 277: 11–18

Beard R W, Turner R C, Oakley N 1971 Fetal response to glucose loading. Fetal blood glucose and insulin responses to hyperglycaemia in normal and diabetic pregnancies. Postgraduate Medical Journal 47: 68–70

Bleicher S J, O'Sullivan J B, Freinkel N 1964 Carbohydrate metabolism in pregnancy. V. The interrelation of glucose, insulin and free fatty acids in late pregnancy and post partum. New England Journal of Medicine 271: 866–872

Burke C W, Roulet F 1970 Increased exposure of the tissues to cortisol in late pregnancy. British Medical Journal 1: 657–659

Burt R L 1956 Peripheral utilisation of insulin in pregnancy and the puerperium. Obstetrics and Gynaecology 2: 658–664

Costrini N V, Kalkhoff R K 1971 Relative effects of pregnancy estradiol and progesterone on plasma insulin and pancreatic islet insulin secretion. Journal of Clinical Investigation 50: 992–999

Davison J M 1974 Changes in renal function and other aspects of homeostasis in early pregnancy. Journal of Obstetrics and Gynaecology of the British Commonwealth 81: 1003–1006

Davison J M, Hytten F E 1975 Renal handling of glucose in pregnancy. In: Sutherland H W, Stowers J M (eds). Carbohydrate metabolism in pregnancy and the newborn. Churchill Livingstone, London, pp 2–17

Fischer P M, Hamilton P M, Sutherland H W et al 1974 The effect of gestation on intravenous glucose tolerance in women. Journal of Obstetrics and Gynaecology of the British Commonwealth 81: 285–290

Flint D J, Sinnett-Smith P A, Clegg R A, Vernon R G 1979 Role of insulin receptors in the changing metabolism of adipose tissue during pregnancy and lactation in the rat. Biochemical Journal 182: 421–427

Gemzell C A 1953 Blood levels of 17 hydroxy corticosteroids in normal pregnancy. Journal of Clinical Endocrinology 13: 898–902

Goldstein R, Levy E, Shafrir E 1985 Increased maternal-fetal transport of fat in diabetes assessed by the polyunsaturated fatty acid content in fetal fluids. Biology of the Neonate 47 (6): 343–349

Green I C, Taylor K W 1972 Effects of pregnancy in the rat on the size and insulin secretory response of the Islets of Langerhan. Journal of Endocrinology 54: 317–325

Hagin A 1961 lslet cell adenoma without symptoms during pregnancy. Nord Medicine 66: 1032–1035

Hellman B 1960 The islets of Langerhans in the rat during pregnancy and lactation with special reference to the changes in the B/A ratio. Acta Obstetrica et Gynecologica Scandinavia 39: 331–349

Kalkhoff R, Kissebah A H, Hak Joong K 1979 Lipid metabolism during normal pregnancy. In: Merkatz K R, Adam P A J (eds) The diabetic pregnancy; a perinatal perspective. Grune and Stratton, New York, pp 10–17

Khan C R 1978 Insulin resistance, insulin insensitivity and insulin responsiveness: a necessary distinction. Metabolism 27: Suppl 2: 1893–1902

Luyckx A S, Gerard J, Gaspard U et al 1975 Plasma glucagon levels in normal women during pregnancy. Diabetologia 11: 549–554

Kühl C 1975 Glucose metabolism during and after pregnancy in normal and gestational diabetic women. Acta Endocrinology 75: 709–719

Lind T, Hytten F E 1972 The excretion of glucose during normal pregnancy. Journal of Obstetrics and Gynaecology of the British Commonwealth 79: 961–964

Lind T, Billewicz W Z, Brown G 1973 A serial study of changes in oral glucose tolerance in pregnancy. Journal of Obstetrics and Gynaecology of the British Commonwealth 80: 1033–1039

Metzger B E, Freinkel N 1975 Regulation of protein metabolism and gluconeogenesis in the fasted state. In: Comerini-Davalos R A, Cole H S (eds) Early diabetes in early life. Academic Press, New York, pp 303–312

Moore P, Kolterman O, Weymart J, Glefoky J M 1981 Insulin binding in human pregnancy. Comparisons to the post partum, luteal and follicular states. Journal of Clinical Endocrinology and Metabolism 52: 937–941

Oakley N W, Beard R W, Turner R C 1972 Effect of sustained maternal hyperglycaemia on the fetus in normal and diabetic pregnancies. British Medical Journal 1: 466–468

O'Sullivan G C, Walker K, Bondar G F 1975 Effects of pregnancy on bile acid metabolism. Surgical Forum 26: 442–444

Pedersen J 1977 The pregnant diabetic and her newborn. Williams and Wilkins, Baltimore Md, pp 24–32

Pedersen O, Beck Nielsen H, Klebe J G 1981 Insulin receptors in the pregnant diabetic and her newborn. Journal of Clinical Endocrinology and Metabolism 53: 1160–1166

Puavilai G, Drobny E C, Damont L A, Baumann G 1982 Insulin receptors and insulin resistance in human pregnancy: evidence for post receptor effect in insulin action. Journal of Clinical Endocrinology and Metabolism 54: 247–252

Ryan M J, Meigs R, Petro Z 1966 The formation of progesterone by the human placenta. American Journal of Obstetrics and Gynaecology 96: 676–686

Telgedy G, Weeks J W, Archer D F et al 1962. Acetate and cholesterol metabolism in the human feto-placental unit at mid gestation. 3. Steroids synthesised and secreted by the fetus. Acta Endocrinology and Metabolism 22: 134–141

Tsiblis J C M, Raynor L O, Buhi W C, Baggie J, Spellacy W N 1980 Insulin receptors in circulating erythrocytes and monocytes from women on oral contraceptives or pregnant women near term. Journal of Clinical Endocrinology and Metabolism 51: 711–717

Tyson J E, Hwang P, Guyda H et al 1972 Studies of prolactin secretion in human pregnancy. American Journal of Obstetrics and Gynaecology 113: 14–20

Ursell W, Brudenell M, Chard T 1973 Placental lactogen levels in diabetic pregnancy. British Medical Journal 2: 80–82

Victor A 1974 Normal blood sugar variation during pregnancy. Acta Obstetrica et Gynecologica Scandinavia 53: 37–40

3
Glycosylated haemoglobin

Haemoglobin A (HbA) constitutes 90% of the haemoglobin found in the red cells of adults and infants over the age of 6 months. Haemoglobin A_1 results from glycosylation of HbA during the lifetime of the red cell.

Glycosylation of haemoglobin occurs as a two-stage process. The first is a rapid and reversible non-enzymatic attachment between the glucose molecule and the N-terminal amino group of the beta haemoglobin molecule (Schiff base linkage) and to a lesser extent the N-terminal groups in the alpha chains and the E-amino group of lysine residues of both alpha and beta chains (Gabbay et al 1979). The second is the Amadori rearrangement leading to the formation of a stable ketoamine linkage HbA_1. HbA_1 is subdivided into HbA_{1a1}, HbA_{1a2}, HbA_{1b} and HbA_{1c}. Of these, HbA_{1c} is the most important and accounts for 4% of the total haemoglobin. The level of HbA_1 is dependent upon the mean level of blood glucose and is raised in diabetics. During rapid changes of diabetic control, the labile fraction, which is thought to be the Schiff base, reflects transient rather than the long-term changes which occur throughout the life of the red cell. The value of HbA_1 (or HbA_{1c}) measurements on the maternal blood in diabetic pregnancy is that it gives an indication of the level of blood glucose during the preceding 4–6 weeks. In normal pregnancy, HbA_1 levels are unchanged or slightly low.

HbA_1 has been found to increase in anaemia in the absence of haemolysis (Brooks et al 1980) and to be decreased in chronic renal failure (Dandona et al 1979). The latter is probably related to the shortened lifespan of erythrocytes, so that those in circulation have a relatively short time to glycosylate haemoglobin. The same applies to haemolytic disease. The methods for measurement of glycosylated haemoglobin include ion exchange chromatography (Kynoch & Lehmann 1977), affinity chromatography (Hall et al 1980), isoelectric focussing (Welinder & Svensen 1980), high pressure liquid chromatography (Cole et al 1978) and colorimetric assay (Gabbay et al 1979). All methods in modern use should include elimination of the labile fraction. This can be achieved by saline incubation or dialysis, leaving only the stable fraction to be measured (Goldstein et al 1980, Svendsen et al 1980).

A method employing electrophoresis devised by Corning is currently being used in the Diabetic Department in King's College Hospital. It gives a range of 4–8% for non-diabetic individuals. The range is similar to the macro-column ion exchange chromatography method previously used, where it was found that well-controlled pregnant diabetic patients had a mean level of 9.5% and poorly controlled pregnant diabetic patients had a mean level of 15.6% (Leslie et al 1978). During pregnancy, better control of maternal diabetes leads to a progressive fall in HbA$_1$ levels (Fig. 3.1). The level often rises post partum when

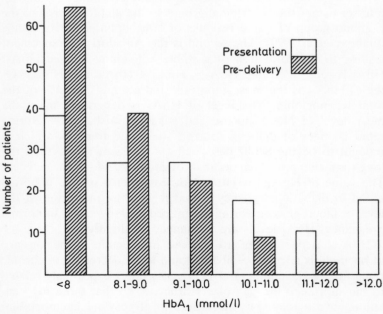

Fig. 3.1 King's College Hospital: HbA$_1$ in diabetic pregnancy 1982–85

the patient is less motivated to continue very careful control (Leslie et al 1978, .Ylinen et al 1981b). This rise does not appear to be related to breastfeeding.

Haemoglobin A₁ and congenital abnormality

Congenital abnormality remains an important cause of perinatal mortality in diabetic pregnancy. Experimental evidence in rats (Deuchar 1979, Eriksson et al 1985) has pointed to an association between maternal hyperglycaemia and congenital abnormality. Mills et al (1979) have emphasized that in human pregnancy hyperglycaemia is most likely to cause malformation during the first 7 weeks when organogenesis is proceeding rapidly. Since glycosylated haemoglobin measurement in the first trimester will give an assessment of diabetic control retrospectively at this crucial time in development, various studies have examined HbA_1 at this stage. It was observed (Leslie et al 1978) that three out of five women with high glycosylated haemoglobin measurements at presentation had babies with congenital malformations, including hemivertebrae, neural tube defects and congenital heart disease. This led to a multicentre trial in the United Kingdom (Stubbs et al 1987). Out of 230 diabetic pregnancies in 196 women there were 7 (3%) major and 21 (9%) minor malformations. The median HbA_1 of those with major malformations (12.9%) was significantly greater than the median HbA_1 of those with no malformations (10.8%). The median HbA_1 of those with minor malformations (10.5%) was not significantly different from those that did not have such malformations. These findings are in accord with the experience at King's College Hospital. Of 6 major malformations in the years 1981–85, 5 were associated

Table 3.1 HbA_1 in first trimester and major congenital malformations: King's College Hospital 1981–85

HbA_1 %	Congenital malformations
8.9	Microcephaly
11.0	Absent radius, deformed thumbs Hemivertebrae
11.6	Caudal regression
12.3	Truncus ateriosus
12.4	Microcephaly
13.8	Multiple (including exomphalos)

with a raised HbA_1 level (Table 3.1). Three other centres have assessed the incidence of congenital abnormalities with respect to diabetic control in the first trimester. Miller et al (1981) at the Joslin Clinic in America, in a retrospective series, found that in the period 1977–80, 116 insulin-dependent diabetic women were seen in the first 14 weeks of gestation: the incidence of major anomalies was 22.4% in 58 infants of women with an initial HbA_1 above 8.5%, whereas it was 3.4% in 58 infants of infants with an initial HbA_1 below 8.5%. Ylinen et al (1984), in Finland, looked at 142 pregnancies from 1978 to 1982 between the 6th and 15th weeks of gestation and found major malformations in 2 out of 63 pregnancies (3.2%) with initial HbA_1 values below 8%, 5 out of 62 pregnancies (8%) with initial HbA_1 values of 8.0–9.0% and four out of 17 pregnancies (23.5%) with initial HbA_1 values above 10%. Fuhrmann et al (1983), in the German Democratic Republic, studied 420 deliveries from 1977 to 1981 but did not record HbA_1 values for these. In contrast to these findings Mills et al (1988) could find no relationship between glycaemic control during organogenesis in diabetic pregnancy and congenital malformation. Raised glucose and glycosylated haemoglobin levels did not occur more frequently in women who had abnormal babies. However, in their series those diabetic women who were seen within 21 days of conception had a lower incidence of malformation than those who were seen later, justifying the attempt to achieve good control around the time of conception.

Haemoglobin A₁ and spontaneous abortion

The trial by Stubbs et al (1987) quoted above showed no relationship between miscarriage and HbA_1 levels. Other studies by Wright et al (1983) and Miodovnik (1984) have reported high rates of miscarriage in diabetic pregnancy—26% and 30%, respectively. In the former study HbA_1 levels were found to be higher in those women who aborted spontaneously.

Cord blood HbA₁

HbF can interfere with results, except when the colorimetric method is used (Pecoraro et al 1979). Its assay in cord blood using ion exchange chromatography (Schwartz 1980, Fadel et al

1981) and isoelectric focussing probably measures both glycosylated and acetylated HbF. Radioimmunoassay has been used to measure HbA_1 in cord blood and more recently affinity chromatography (Hall et al 1980). This method, with minor modifications, has the added advantage of determining glycosylated plasma protein in adult and fetal blood as well. Since glycosylation of protein occurs over a shorter time span (10 days to 3 weeks) (Kennedy & Baynes 1984), this may prove to be a more sensitive indicator of changes in overall control. Fructosamine, a measure of serum glycosylated proteins, correlates significantly with glycosylated haemoglobin (Baker et al 1983) and is currently being evaluated in pregnancy.

Cord blood glycosylated haemoglobin levels are higher in infants of diabetic mothers compared with infants of non-diabetic mothers and consistently lower in cord blood than maternal blood for both groups (Sosenko et al 1982, Worth et al 1983). Cord glycosylated haemoglobin values were significantly increased in diabetic babies who developed hypoglycaemia (Worth et al 1983). Neonatal hypoglycaemia has been associated with a raised maternal HbA_1 value in both the second and third trimesters and neonatal hyperbilirubinaemia with a raised HbA_1 in the third trimester. A raised maternal HbA_1 value in the second trimester was also associated significantly with a higher incidence of perinatal death (Ylinen, Raivio & Teramo 1981a).

Maternal HbA_1 correlation with birthweight

Birthweight ratio (birthweight divided by the 50th centile birthweight for gestational age) did not correlate with cord or maternal HbA_1 at delivery in one series (Worth et al 1983) and was explained by relatively 'tight' control of maternal diabetes towards the end of pregnancy. There have been conflicting reports about the correlation of maternal HbA_1 with birthweight or birthweight ratio. O'Shaughnessy et al (1979), Stubbs et al (1981), Fadel et al (1981), Miller et al (1981), Poon et al (1981) and Sosenko et al (1982) did not find such a correlation but others have found a link between third trimester HbA_1 and relative birthweight (Widness et al 1978, Ylinen et al 1981). Knight (1983) and Russell (1984) found near-normal HbA_1 levels in macrosomic pregnancy.

Conclusion

HbA$_1$ levels are of considerable value during pregnancy and form a logical part of prepregnancy counselling. The level of HbA$_1$ in the first trimester identifies those diabetic pregnancies most likely to be associated with congenital malformations. Levels of HbA$_1$ above normal during the latter part of pregnancy indicate that greater attention needs to be given to the patient's diabetic control and may give a warning of developing macrosomia. The post partum HbA$_1$ level may be of value as a screen for unrecognized gestational diabetes where there has been macrosomia or unexplained late intrauterine fetal death (Steel et al 1981, Widness et al 1981).

REFERENCES

Baker J R, O'Connor J P, Metcalf P A, Lawson M R, Johnson R N 1983 Clinical usefulness of estimation of serum fructosamine concentration as a screening test for diabetes mellitus. British Medical Journal 287: 863–867

Brooks A P, Metcalfe J, Day J L, Edwards M S 1980 Iron deficiency and glycosylated haemoglobin A$_1$. Lancet ii: 141

Cole R A, Solender J S, Dunn P J, Bunn H F 1978 A rapid method for the determination of glycosylated haemoglobins using high pressure liquid chromatography. Metabolism 27: 289–301

Dandona P, Freedman D, Moorhead F J 1979 Glycosylated haemoglobin in chronic renal failure. British Medical Journal i: 1183–1184

Deuchar E M 1979 Experimental evidence relating fetal abnormalities to diabetes. In: Sutherland H W, Stowers J M (eds) Carbohydrate metabolism in pregnancy and the newborn. Springer Verlag, Berlin, 49: 519–522

Eriksson U J, Dahlstrom E, Hellerstrom C 1985 Metabolically determined teratogenesis: malformations and maternal diabetes. Biochemical Society Transactions 13: 79–82

Fadel H E, Reynolds A, Stallings M, Abraham E C 1981 Minor (glycosylated) hemoglobins in cord blood of infants of normal and diabetic mothers. Journal of Obstetrics and Gynaecology 139: 397–402

Fuhrmann K, Reiher H, Semmler K et al 1983 Prevention of congenital malformations in infants of insulin-dependent diabetic mothers. Diabetes Care 6: 219–223.

Gabbay K H, Sosenko J M, Banuchi C A, Mininsohn M J, Fluckiger R 1979. Glycosylated hemoglobins: increased glycosylation of hemoglobin A in diabetic patients. Diabetes 28: 337–340

Goldstein D E, Peth S B, England J D, Hess R L, DaCosta J 1980 Effects of acute changes in blood glucose on HbA$_{1c}$. Diabetes 29: 623–628

Hall P M, Cawdell G M, Cook J G H, Gould B J 1980 Measurement of glycosylated haemoglobins and glycosylated plasma proteins in maternal and cord blood using an affinity chromatography method. Diabetologia 19: 477–487

Kennedy L, Baynes J W 1984 Non-enzymatic glycosylation and the chronic complications of diabetes; an overview. Diabetologia 98: 93–98

Knight A 1983 Concerning macrosomy in diabetic pregnancy. Lancet ii: 1431

Kynoch P A M, Lehmann H 1977 Rapid estimation (2 1/2 hours) of glycosylated haemoglobin for routine purposes. Lancet ii: 16

Leslie R D G, Pyke D A, John P N, White J M 1978 Haemoglobin A_1 in diabetic pregnancy. Lancet ii: 958–959

Miller E, Hare J W, Cloherty J P et al 1981 Elevated maternal haemoglobin A_{1c} in early pregnancy and major congenital anomalies in infants of diabetic mothers. New England Journal of Medicine 304: 1331–1334

Mills J L, Baker L, Goldman A S 1979 Malformations in infants of diabetic mothers occur before the seventh gestational week. Diabetes 28: 292–293

Mills J L, Knopp R H, Simpson J L et al 1988 Lack of relation of increased malformation rates in infants of diabetic mothers to glycaemia control during organogenesis. New England Journal of Medicine 318: 671–676

Miodovnik M, Lavin J P, Knowles H C et al 1984 Spontaneous abortion among insulin-dependent diabetic women. American Journal of Obstetrics and Gynecology 150 (4): 372–376

O'Shaughnessy R, Cuss J, Zuspan F P 1979 Glycosylated hemoglobins and diabetes mellitus in pregnancy. American Journal of Obstetrics and Gynecology 135: 783–790

Pecoraro R E, Graf R J, Halter J B, Beiter H, Porte D 1979 Comparison of a colorimetric assay for glycosylated hemoglobin with ion-exchange chromatography. Diabetes 28: 1120–1125

Poon P, Turner R C, Gillmer M D G 1981 Glycosylated fetal haemoglobin. British Medical Journal 283: 469

Russell G, Farmer G, Lloyd D et al 1984 Macrosomia despite well-controlled diabetic pregnancy. Lancet 1: 283–284

Schwartz H C, Widness J, Thompson D, Tsubol K K et al 1980 Glycosylation and acetylation of haemoglobin in infants of normal and diabetic mothers. Biology of the Neonate 38: 71–75

Sosenko J M, Kitzmiller J L, Fluckiger R et al 1982 Umbilical cord Glycosylated hemoglobin in infants of diabetic mothers: relationship to neonatal hypoglycaemia macrosomia and cord serum C-peptide. Diabetes Care 5: 566–570

Steel J M, Thomson P, Johnstone F et al 1981 Glycosylated haemoglobin concentrations in mothers of large babies. British Medical Journal 282: 1357–1358

Stubbs S M, Leslie R D G, John P N 1981 Fetal macrosomia and maternal diabetic control in pregnancy. British Medical Journal 282: 439–440

Stubbs S M, Doddridge M, John P N, Steel J M, Wright A D 1987 Haemoglobin A_1 and congenital malformations. Diabetic Medicine 4: 156–159

Svendsen P Aa, Christiansen J S, Soegaard U, Welinder B S, Nerup J 1980. Rapid changes in chromatographically determined haemoglobin A_{1c} induced by short term changes in glucose concentration. Diabetologia 19: 130–136

Welinder B S, Svendsen P Aa 1980 Heterogeneity of the haemoglobin-A_{1c}-bond in isoelectric focussing. Diabetologia 19: 465–467

Widness J A, Schwartz H C, Thompson D et al 1978. Haemoglobin A_{1c} (glycohaemoglobin) in diabetic pregnancy: an indicator of glucose control and fetal size. British Journal of Obstetrics and Gynaecology 85: 812–817

Widness J A, Schwartz H C, Zeller W P, Ott W, Schwartz R 1981 Glycohaemoglobin in postpartum women. Obstetrics and Gynecology 57: 414–421.

Worth R, Ashworth L, Home P et al 1983 Glycosylated haemoglobin in cord blood following normal and diabetic pregnancies. Diabetologia 25(6): 482–485

Wright A D, Nicholson H O, Pollock A, Taylor K G, Betts S 1983
Spontaneous abortion and diabetes mellitus. Postgraduate Medical Journal
59: 295–298

Ylinen K, Raivio K, Teramo K 1981 (a) Haemoglobin A_{1c} predicts the
perinatal outcome in insulin dependent diabetic pregnancies. British Journal
of Obstetrics and Gynaecology 88: 961–967

Ylinen K, Hekali R, Teramo K 1981 (b) Haemoglobin A_{1c} during pregnancy of
insulin dependent diabetics and healthy controls. Journal of Obstetrics and
Gynecology 1: 223–228

Ylinen K, Aula P, Stenman U-H et al 1984 Risk of minor and major fetal
malformations in diabetics with high haemoglobin A_{1c} values in early
pregnancy. British Medical Journal 289: 345–346

4

Preconception care

The mainstay of the management of the pregnant diabetic is good diabetic control: it is logical for the diabetic woman who plans to become pregnant to ensure that her diabetes is as well controlled as she and her diabetic physician can make it. The importance of good control during the first trimester especially relates to the occurrence of congenital abnormality (see Ch 7). For the diabetic woman with vascular complications it is also important that she discuss fully the implications of pregnancy and, in the case of retinopathy, have any appropriate treatment.

At King's College Hospital the clinical notes of all diabetic women between the ages of 16 and 40 are marked with a green sticker. At their initial visit they are asked if they are planning a pregnancy at some stage in the future. If the answer is 'no', 'no further pregnancy is planned' is entered into the patient's notes alongside the green sticker. Such patients are offered family planning advice or, in some cases, sterilization as appropriate. If the answer is 'yes', the importance of good control in all stages of pregnancy is discussed with the patient and she is asked to attend the clinic 3 months before she starts to try to become pregnant for a 'preconception check up'. This consists of:

1. complete physical examination to confirm fitness for pregnancy;
2. intensified blood glucose tests;
3. HbA$_1$ estimation

If the results of (2) and (3) are abnormal, appropriate adjustments are made to diet and insulin regimen.

4. Any patient who is not already doing home monitoring of blood glucose levels is encouraged to do so using either a glucose oxidase strip alone or with a glucose meter. The results obtained are recorded and kept for the next diabetic clinic visit which should be no longer than 3 months.

The obstetrician's contribution to preconception care

It is very helpful for the obstetrician to see these patients. Any anxieties they may have about pregnancy should be discussed and, in the case of multigravidas, the past obstetric history carefully reviewed. The importance of keeping a menstrual calendar should be emphasized so that the pregnancy can be accurately dated. When infertility is a problem suitable investigations should be undertaken. The rubella status, blood pressure and weight should be checked and the patient who smokes should be discouraged from doing so.

Advantages of preconception care

Most women welcome the opportunity to discuss planning for pregnancy. By using appropriate contraception, the number of unplanned pregnancies can be reduced and accordingly the number of women who go through the first trimester without special attention to diabetic control reduced. Perhaps the greatest value of the preconception approach is that it motivates the patient to manage her general health and diabetes in a way most likely to lead to a successful pregnancy. At the present time, 30% of all women attending the diabetic antenatal clinic at King's College Hospital have had preconception care. The proportion of those who regularly attend the King's diabetic clinic is higher. It is hard to quantify the advantages claimed but the strong impression is that those who have had such care do better in pregnancy. Steel (1985) reports that in Edinburgh 74% of the regular attenders at the diabetic clinic attend the pre-pregnancy clinic. There was a higher incidence of congenital abnormality in those who did not attend. This is probably due to the fact that the non-attenders were more likely to be poorly motivated and consequently badly controlled. Goldman et al (1986) compared the outcome in 44 women with IDD who attended a preconception clinic with 31 who did not. The latter group had a higher incidence of maternal complications such as pre-eclampsia. There were three congenital malformations in the offspring of the non-attenders, compared with none in those of the preconception care group. Fuhrman et al (1983) has reported a significant reduction in congenital abnormality, from 7.5% in 292 diabetics seen after eight weeks of gestation to 0.8% in 128 diabetics seen whilst planning a pregnancy. Jensen et al (1986) used the continuous subcutaneous route for insulin administration in nine patients for at least two months prior to conception. Better metabolic control was achieved than in 11 control patients treated with intermittent injections, but there was no difference in the clinical outcome, which was equally good in both groups. Preconception care is a most important aspect of the management of diabetic pregnancy and holds out the best hope for reducing the number of congenital abnormalities.

REFERENCES

Fuhrman K, Reiher H, Semmer K, Fischer F, Fischer M, Glockner E 1983 Prevention of congenital malformations in infants of insulin dependent diabetic mothers. Diabetes Care 6: 219–223

Goldman J A, Dicker D, Feldberg D, Yeshaya A, Samuel N, Karp M 1986 Pregnancy outcome in patients with insulin dependent diabetes mellitus with preconception diabetic control: a comparative study. American Journal of Obstetrics and Gynecology 155: 293–297

Jensen B M, Kuhl C, Mølsted-Pedersen L, Saurbreg N, Fog-Pedersen J 1986 Preconception treatment with insulin infusion pumps in insulin dependent diabetic women with particular reference to the prevention of congenital malformations. Acta Endocrinologica Supplement (Copenhagen) 277: 81–85

Steel J M 1985 The pre-pregnancy clinic. Practical Diabetes 2(6): 8–10

5

Antenatal screening

The alternations in carbohydrate metabolism, in particular the increased need for insulin in pregnancy, result in a small proportion of women becoming diabetic or at least developing impaired glucose tolerance during the course of pregnancy. The definition of gestational diabetes (GDM) and of impaired glucose tolerance (IGT) in pregnancy is considered in Chapter 2. The distinction between the two conditions is not academic, although they represent different degrees of the same change and the one, impaired glucose tolerance, precedes the other. The development of impaired glucose tolerance or gestational diabetes is most likely to occur toward the end of the second trimester or during the third trimester. This is the time at which insulin antagonists such as human placental lactogen are at their highest concentration and the resistance to insulin correspondingly increased (Ursell et al 1973). The importance of detecting a change in the pregnant woman's carbohydrate metabolism relates particularly to gestational diabetes, for if this condition is not recognized and treated the consequences for the fetus may be serious.

Perinatal mortality in undetected gestational diabetes occurs either because of the classic complications of diabetic pregnancy, particularly late unexplained intrauterine death, or profound neonatal hyperglycaemia. The way in which gestational diabetes is detected is by clinical observation and simple urine testing or by applying a specific screening test to the whole antenatal population. Patients who develop gestational diabetes will, eventually, have the symptoms of diabetes especially thirst and polyuria and will also show glycosuria and ketonuria. In the early stages of the condition, however, such symptoms may be mild and overlooked or attributed to pregnancy. Glycosuria and ketonuria are likely to be intermittent and may, therefore, escape detection. The lack of a constant relationship between hyperglycaemia and glycosuria in pregnancy increases the difficulty. The presence of hydramnios or the development of fetal macrosomia should always alert the obstetrician: both call for an estimation of maternal blood glucose levels.

The alternative to clinical detection of gestational diabetes is antenatal screening, and a great deal of interest and effort has centred on finding an ideal screening method. Although glycosuria and ketonuria are unreliable as routine tests for gestational diabetes they do, nevertheless, provide a crude test for the condition, especially when glycosuria appears early in the pregnancy (before the 20th week) or is persistent and heavy later on. Glycosuria and ketonuria together are diagnostic of diabetes in most cases, so that a simple test for ketone bodies in urine showing heavy glycosuria will pick up some of the women whose glycosuria is not simply the result of altered renal handling of glucose in pregnancy. It must, however, be accepted that gestational diabetes may develop without glycosuria being detected by routine antenatal clinic testing, especially as many women attending antenatal clinics bring the first early morning specimen of urine which is the least likely to be positive for glucose. Impaired glucose tolerance cannot be diagnosed clinically and is even less likely to be detected by urine testing. Whether or not this condition is significant per se is debatable (see Ch. 2) but it may progress to gestational diabetes later in the pregnancy and there is no argument about the importance of this latter condition.

Specific antenatal screening tests for impaired glucose tolerance and gestational diabetes

The problem with screening tests in pregnancy is that they tend to be time consuming and expensive. Their use can only be justified if they have a significant detection rate. On this ground antenatal screening tests for diabetes can be justified if resources permit, but they are not likely to make a big impact on perinatal mortality and morbidity rates, since the incidence of otherwise undetected gestational diabetes is likely to be small. The object of the screening test is to detect asymptomatic gestational diabetes and women with impaired glucose tolerance. Because of the unreliability of urinary glucose estimations and the traditional stigmata of potential diabetes as pointers to impaired glucose tolerance (IGT) or GDM, a screening test should be based on blood glucose estimation.

The most effective screening test is a full glucose tolerance test (GTT) at or about 30 weeks, but this would be too costly and time consuming in practice. A random blood glucose estimation, on the other hand, is simple and may easily be combined with other routine antenatal blood tests. Allowance must be made when interpreting the results of random testing for the time of the last meal. Lind & Anderson (1984) adopted such a screening test, dividing the patients up into two groups, those who had eaten within 2 hours of the blood sample being taken and those who had had their last meal more than 2 hours previously. A blood glucose level of 6.4 mmol/l or more for the former, or 5.8 mmol/l for the latter, was taken as indicating the need for a full oral glucose tolerance test. About 1% of the antenatal population were picked out by these criteria at 28 weeks and of these about half had some impairment of glucose tolerance with the full oral GTT. The American National Diabetes Data Group (1979), suggesting a similar approach, used plasma glucose levels of 5.8 mmol/l or more random fasting and 6.7 mmol/l or more random post-prandial to indicate the need for a full oral GTT.

The O'Sullivan & Mahan (1964) screening test, using blood glucose estimations on whole blood, measures the level 1 hour after oral ingestion of 50 g glucose. A level of greater than 8.3 mmol/l is taken to be positive and the full GTT is then carried out. Gillmer et al (1980), using the same glucose load, suggested 7.7 mmol/l as the critical level. They screened all patients in one antenatal clinic for 1 year by estimating plasma glucose 1 hour after oral ingestion of 50 g glucose and, taking a plasma glucose level of greater than 7.7 mmol/l, identified 74 out

Table 5.1 Screening for gestational diabetes and impaired glucose tolerance

Random test (mmol/l glucose)	Pre-prandial	Post-prandial
US NDD group (plasma)	≥ 5.8	≥ 6.7
Lind (venous blood)	≥ 5.8	≥ 6.4
50 g oral glucose load		1 hour level
O'Sullivan (venous blood)		≥ 8.3
Gillmer (venous plasma)		≥ 7.7
Landon et al (capillary blood)		≥ 8.9

of 948 women. Sixty-eight of these women were given an oral GTT and 14 (1.5% of the study population) were found to have IGT. Nine of the 14 had one or more of the screening criteria shown in Table 5.2. It is worth pointing out that Gillmer used a 50 g glucose load when carrying out the full oral GTT and not the presently recommended 75 g load.

A more recent study (Marquette, Klein & Miebyl 1985) followed the O'Sullivan/Gillmer technique; a cut-off point of 7.2 mmol/l resulted, after GTT testing, in a 2.4% incidence of impaired glucose tolerance in those women without classical risk factors and a 3.3% incidence of those with these factors. In evaluating the cost effectiveness of this method of screening, the authors point out that screening on the basis of risk factors alone is inefficient. However, if only those patients who are 24 or older are screened the cost is halved without much loss of sensitivity (10 out of 12 detected cases were aged 24 or more).

Landon et al (1986) used a simple glucose reflectance meter in the antenatal clinic to measure the capillary blood glucose level after a 50 g oral glucose load between 26 and 28 weeks' gestation. A glucose level at 1 hour of 8.9 mmol/l (160 mg%) or more was taken as an indication for a full oral GTT. They concluded that this method was a cheap and effective way of screening for gestational diabetes.

When glycosylated haemoglobin was introduced into the management of diabetes it was hoped that it would be an ideal screening method for GDM. Sadly, this has not proved to be the case, for although there is a correlation between mean blood glucose levels and HbA_1 levels the sensitivity of the method is not high enough to be useful (Artal et al 1984). The most useful application of HbA_1 estimations in this respect is in women who have unexplained macrosomic stillbirths. A post-partum oral GTT is of little use in such cases, but a raised HbA_1 level suggests that the woman may have had undiagnosed gestational diabetes during the pregnancy.

Roberts & Baker (1986) have reported on the measurement of serum fructosamine levels as a screening test for diabetes in pregnancy. They found a good correlation between fructosamine levels and the oral GTT. A serum fructosamine greater than the 95th percentile was found in 8 of 9 women who had gestational diabetes diagnosed by glucose tolerance testing. The authors feel that the estimation of serum fructosamine may be a useful screening test, but greater experience of the method is needed before it can be recommended as an alternative to glucose tolerance testing.

Clearly, no method of screening for impairment of carbohydrate metabolism in pregnancy is entirely satisfactory. Clinicians running busy antenatal clinics may feel unable to add to the load of clinic staff by instituting an additional blood test or tests. In such situations reliance must be placed on the detection of glycosuria, clinical symptoms of diabetes, hydramnios and excessive fetal growth, especially in the last trimester. Blood glucose measurements are reserved for these 'suspicious' cases. This approach will, however, fail to detect most cases of impaired glucose tolerance and up to 50% of women with true gestational diabetes (Gabbe 1985).

The screening tests listed in Table 5.1 are likely to pick out between 1 and 1.5% of the population screened as having some degree of impaired glucose tolerance. Whether this will significantly affect a unit's overall perinatal mortality or morbidity will depend on the general standards of antenatal, intrapartum and paediatric neonatal care. Where these standards are high the impact will probably be negligible. Mølsted-Pedersen (1984), in describing the Copenhagen model of practical screening, which is based on clinical criteria (family history, overweight by 20% just before pregnancy, previous heavy baby of 4.5 kg or more) and glycosuria as indications for an oral GTT, found an incidence of 1% gestational diabetes. He concluded that if these criteria were used throughout Denmark, some 20% of stillbirths from this cause could be avoided per annum. This estimate was arrived at on the basis that only 15% of all gestational diabetics are currently diagnosed and that the perinatal mortality rate of the undiagnosed is 40. Since the Copenhagen criteria are probably the most commonly used in the UK, some comfort can be taken that not many cases of gestational diabetes leading to perinatal mortality will be missed. Many clinicians will, however, wish to

Table 5.2 Clinical criteria for doing a glucose tolerance test

1. Potential diabetics (family history, previous heavy baby)
2. Obesity: over 20% of ideal weight for height
3. Glycosuria on two or more occasions, especially if the morning post-prandial specimen examined
4. Previous congenital abnormality, unexplained stillbirth or neonatal death
5. Hydramnios in current pregnancy
6. Previous gestational diabetes
7. Developing fetal macrosomia

employ some method of antenatal screening for carbohydrate intolerance and should use either random or post-glucose load blood glucose estimations, depending on their available resources. The simplest and cheapest approach is to do a random blood glucose estimation between 28 and 30 weeks and define a level in the population being screened above which an oral GTT will be performed. This level will probably be between 2 and 3 standard deviations above the mean random level. Lind's method is an example of how this screening test can be applied in practice, and if used at 28–30 weeks only is unlikely to impose too great a burden on even the busiest antenatal clinic staff, whilst at the same time detecting a majority of women showing impaired glucose tolerance and all true gestational diabetics. If economies have to be made in even such a simple screening method then excluding those under 25 years old is reasonable and will only result in a very few cases being missed. Ultimately, the yardstick by which the need for routine antenatal testing must be measured from an obstetric view point is whether or not it significantly affects perinatal outcome and maternal health. The balance of evidence has now shifted towards the use of some form of screening test of maternal blood glucose levels.

REFERENCES

Artal R, Mosley G M, Dorey F J 1984 Glycohaemoglobin as a screening test for gestational diabetes. American Journal of Obstetrics and Gynecology 148: 412–414

Gabbe S G 1985 Management of diabetes mellitus in pregnancy. American Journal of Obstetrics and Gynecology 153 (2): 824–828

Gillmer M D G, Oakley N W, Beard R W et al 1980 Antenatal screening for diabetes mellitus by random blood glucose sampling. British Journal of Obstetrics and Gynaecology 87: 377–382

Landon M B, Cernbrowski G S, Gabbe S G 1986 Capillary blood glucose screening for gestational diabetes: a preliminary investigation. American Journal of Obstetrics and Gynecology 155: 717–721

Lind T, Anderson J 1984 Does random blood glucose sampling outdate testing for glycosuria in the detection of diabetes during pregnancy. British Medical Journal 289: 1569–1571

Marquette G P, Klein V R and Miebyl J R 1985 Efficacy of screening for gestational diabetes. American Journal of Perinatology 2(1): 7–9

Mølsted-Pedersen L 1984 Detection of gestational diabetes. In: Sutherland H W, Stowers J M (eds) Carbohydrate metabolism in pregnancy and the newborn. Churchill Livingstone, Edinburgh, pp 209–210

National Diabetes Data Group 1979 Classification and diagnosis of diabetes mellitus and other categories of glucose intolerance. Diabetes 28: 1039–1057

O'Sullivan J M, Mahan C H 1964 Criteria for the oral glucose tolerance test in pregnancy. Diabetes 13: 278

Diabetic pregnancy

Roberts A B, Baker J R 1986 Serum fructosamine: a screening test for diabetes in pregnancy. American Journal of Obstetrics and Gynecology 154 (5): 1027–1030

Ursell W, Brudenell M, Chard T 1973 Placental lactogen levels in diabetic pregnancy. British Medical Journal 2: 80–82

6

Diabetic complications and pregnancy

The effect of diabetic complications on pregnancy outcome

Diabetes is associated with an increased incidence of vascular disease. Diabetic micro- and macroangiopathy develop to a variable extent and over a variable period of time in many diabetics. Diabetic retinopathy is a leading cause of new cases of blindness in women aged 20–74 years in the USA. Lesser degrees of visual impairment are common, although nowadays the numbers of women becoming blind can be reduced by photocoagulation. Diabetic nephropathy, as indicated by persistent proteinuria, is found in approximately 10% of diabetics. The incidence increases with the duration of diabetes and after 15 years one third of insulin-dependent diabetics and one fifth of non-insulin-dependent diabetics will have developed nephropathy (National Diabetic Data Group Report 1984). Peripheral vascular disease and neuropathy are also common in diabetics but tend to develop late and rarely cause clinical problems in pregnant women. The adverse effects which diabetic vascular complications may have on pregnancy outcomes were recognized in the White classification (White 1965). This classification is not used at King's College Hospital (see Ch. 1), where women with either retinopathy or nephropathy are considered as a group under the general heading 'Established Diabetes with Complications' (EDC). Comparison of pregnancy outcome for the fetus in established diabetics with and without complications and with gestational diabetics shows that in recent times, given expert diabetic care, the outcome for the fetus is not much worse (see Table 6.1).

Table 6.1 Pregnancy outcome in gestational diabetics and in established
diabetics with and without complications

KCH diabetic pregnancy 1951–85 Perinatal mortality (%)	1951–70	1971–80	1981–85
GROUP I Gestational	36 (16.6)	66 (1.5)	33 (0.0)
GROUP II Established	639 (15.5)	235 (3.3)	133 (0.0)
GROUP III Established with complications	29 (27.5)	30 (10.1)	27 (7.4)

Perinatal mortality rates
Pregnancy in diabetic women with proteinuria

Grenfell et al (1986a) reported the results of 22 pregnancies in
20 diabetic women with persistent proteinuria seen in the diabetic
pregnancy clinic at King's College Hospital between 1974 and
1984. Only two of the women were non-insulin dependent.
Retinopathy was also present in 19 patients, of whom 8 had
proliferative retinopathy. The past obstetric histories were very
poor, only 15 live births including twins resulting from 44 pregnancies. Of the remaining pregnancies 15 ended in miscarriage,
6 in termination of pregnancy, 7 in stillbirth and 2 in neonatal
death. In the pregnancies managed by the combined team at
King's College Hospital, hypertension was present by the third
trimester in 16 women (72%), with 7 having diastolic pressures
of 100 mmHg or more. Early delivery was common, 11 (50%)
being delivered before 37 weeks, mainly because of increasing
hypertension. The caesarean section rate was high (16/22, 72%)
but the outcome for the fetus was good, with 23 live births,
including one set of twins. The babies were smaller than average,
13/22 (65%) being below the 50th centile. Three women with
proteinuria had babies below the 10th centile. These results,
together with those reported by Kitzmiller et al (1981) and
Jovanovic & Jovanovic (1984), indicate that the outlook for the
fetus in diabetic women with proteinuria is good, providing
hypertension and significant renal impairment are absent at the
outset of the pregnancy. Most patients show an increase in
proteinuria during the pregnancy and have stable or falling

creatinine clearance. These changes return to pre-pregnancy levels after delivery, confirming the generally held belief that pregnancy does not cause a permanent deterioration in renal function or accelerate the progress of the underlying renal disease (Katz et al 1980, Hayslett 1984).

Diabetic pregnancy following renal transplantation

Renal transplantation has become increasingly successful in recent years and with the return of fertility pregnancy becomes a possibility. There have been numerous reports of pregnancies in non-diabetic transplant recipients (Penn et al 1980) but only four reported cases in diabetic recipients. One of these occurred at King's College Hospital (Grenfell et al 1986B). The patient had major microvascular complications and had received a cadaver kidney 1 year prior to becoming pregnant. Following this operation she was treated with cyclosporin A and prednisolone and had excellent renal function. The outcome of the pregnancy was successful in spite of blindness, gangrenous toes, hypertension, cardiac impairment and both sensory and autonomic neuropathy. Renal function remained stable during the pregnancy, but proteinuria increased and at 29 weeks the growth retarded baby was delivered by caesarean section. It weighed 1.1 kg at birth but made successful progress thereafter. Following delivery the patient's hypertension improved, the gangrene resolved and renal function remained stable. Pregnancy following renal transplantation is a possibility which should not be overlooked: it may be successful but is not generally advisable in view of the greatly increased risks of obstetric complications and the long-term maternal morbidity and mortality.

Long-term aspects of diabetic renal disease

In spite of the good fetal results in modern obstetric practice and the lack of evidence that pregnancy causes a deterioration in renal function, the long-term outlook for these women is not good. In the series reported above (Grenfell et al 1986a) one patient died of renal failure 1 year after delivery, one awaiting renal transplantation and two had early renal failure.

These facts must be taken into consideration when counselling diabetic women with proteinuria, and in general pregnancy should be discouraged, especially when there is evidence of renal impairment or significant hypertension. If pregnancy is undertaken close cooperation is needed between obstetrician, diabetic and renal physicians and the patient herself must be prepared to cooperate fully in what is likely to be a very complicated pregnancy.

Diabetic retinopathy

Retinopathy is the most easily documented diabetic vascular lesion and has been extensively studied in relation to pregnancy by a number of authors (Carstenson et al 1982). The prevalence of retinopathy is significantly related to the duration of diabetes; approximately 80% of women with diabetes for more than 20 years had retinopathy. Seven per cent had proliferative retinopathy which deteriorated during pregnancy but showed some improvement post partum. It is important to examine the retina of all pregnant diabetics at regular intervals. Background retinopathy generally follows a benign course during pregnancy and does not require treatment.

The effect of pregnancy on the natural course of diabetic retinopathy was assessed by Moloney & Drury (1982). They found that 62% of pregnant women in their survey had some degree of retinopathy at their first examination in pregnancy and 15% developed it as pregnancy progressed, thereby significantly increasing the prevalence of retinopathy during pregnancy. Apart from a moderate increase in microaneurysms, haemorrhages appeared in just over half of their patients and soft exudates in just over a quarter. Streak or blob haemorrhages increased markedly between the 20th and 28th weeks, while soft exudates appeared by 20 weeks and remained relatively constant for the remainder of the pregnancy. Six months after delivery these changes had regressed. If proliferative retinopathy develops, however, laser treatment should be given.

Although retinopathy is a progressive lesion, most authors do not feel that pregnancy makes any difference to the prognosis. Early onset diabetes is more likely to be complicated by retinopathy if renal function is impaired by nephropathy. Successful renal transplant diminishes the risk of severe retinopathy and blindness in these patients. A condition of acute optic disc oedema in insulin-dependent diabetics during pregnancy has been described but it is rare. No treatment is needed and the condition regresses after delivery (Ward et al 1984).

Ischaemic heart disease

This vascular complication of diabetes in pregnancy carries a high risk of maternal mortality. The number of reports in the literature is small. Reece et al (1976) confirm this view, but report the case of a 32-year-old insulin-dependent diabetic who had persistent angina which was treated by a coronary artery bypass operation. She subsequently became pregnant and despite deterioration of retinopathy and nephropathy was safely delivered by caesarean section at 34 weeks. Both mother and baby survived. The advent of coronary artery bypass surgery has improved the qualitative and quantitative survival of patients with coronary artery disease. The effect of pregnancy on long-term survival is unknown. The wisdom of encouraging any woman with such severe vasculopathy to become pregnant is open to doubt.

REFERENCES

Carstenson L L, Frost-Larsen K, Fugleberg S, Nerup J 1982 Does pregnancy influence the prognosis of uncomplicated IDDM? Diabetes Care 5: 1–5
Grenfell A, Brudenell M, Doddridge M C, Watkins P J 1986a Pregnancy in diabetic women with proteinuria. Quarterly Journal of Medicine 228: 279–386
Grenfell A, Bewick M, Brudenell M, Carr J V, Parsons V, Snowden S, Watkins P J 1986b Diabetic pregnancy following renal transplantation. Diabetic Medicine 3: 177–179
Hare J W, White P 1977 Pregnancy in diabetes complicated by vascular disease. Diabetes 26: 953–955
Hayslett J P 1984 Interaction of renal disease and pregnancy. Kidney International 25: 579–587
Jovanovic R, Jovanovic L 1984 Obstetric management when normoglycaemia is maintained in diabetic pregnant women with vascular compromise. American Journal of Obstetrics and Gynecology 149: 617–623
Katz A L, Davison J M, Hayslett J P 1980 Pregnancy in women with kidney disease. Kidney International 18: 192–206

Diabetic pregnancy

Kitzmiller J L, Brown E R, Phillipe M 1981 Diabetic nephropathy and perinatal outcome. American Journal of Obstetrics and Gynecology 141: 741–751

Moloney J B M, Drury M I 1982 The effect of pregnancy on the natural course of diabetic retinopathy. American Journal of Ophthalmology 93: 745–756

National Diabetes, Data Group 1984 Complication of diabetes. Diabetes in America 1: 3–4

Penn K, Makowski E L, Harris P 1980 Parenthood following renal transplantation. Kidney International 18: 22–233

Reece E A, Eagan J F X, Constan D R, Tamberlain A W, Bates S E, O'Neill R M, Fitzpatrick J G 1986 Coronary artery disease in diabetic pregnancies. American Journal of Obstetrics and Gynecology 154: 150–151

Ward S L, Wood D R, Gilstrop L C, Hauth J C 1984 Pregnancy and acute optic disc oedema in insulin dependent diabetics. Obstetrics and Gynecology 64: 816–818

White P 1965 Pregnancy and diabetes; medical aspects. Medical Clinics of North America 49: 1015

7

Medical management

Medical management of diabetic pregnancy is based on diet alone or diet and insulin, depending on the type of maternal diabetes.

Diet

A proper diet is an essential part of the management of all pregnant diabetic women, including gestational diabetics and those with impaired glucose tolerance (Table 7.1). For the established IDD and NIDD patients adjustments to the pre-pregnancy diet may have to be made in the form of an increased allowance of carbohydrate to meet the extra energy requirements of pregnancy. It is most important that the pregnant woman does not add hunger to the other discomforts of pregnancy, but equally any adjustments to diet must take into account the need for tight blood glucose control. For the NIDD patients who become pregnant and for those whose gestational diabetes is mild dietary measures alone may suffice. For the obese, calorie restriction may be necessary as well as a reappraisal of the carbohydrate content of the diet to include a greater amount of dietary fibre. An increase in dietary fibre appears to exert a flattening effect on the post-prandial rise in blood glucose concentrations (Eastwood et al 1979) by slowing the absorption of carbohydrate from the stomach. Fifty per cent or more of the total energy content should be obtained from carbohydrates, as found in wholemeal bread and wholemeal flour, Weetabix, bran flakes, root vegetables and legumes. There should be a reduction in the fat intake to about 35% of the total energy intake. There should be a decrease in dairy products, including many cheeses (but

Diabetic pregnancy

Table 7.1 Suggested dietary requirements for pregnant diabetics

	Protein	Fat	CHO
IDEAL			
Breakfast			
Weetabix × 2	4		20
Skimmed milk 200 ml	6	1.0	10
Wholemeal bread—2 slices	4		20
Thin spread polyunsat. margarine		10	
Mid-Morning			
Tea with skimmed milk	1.0	—	1.5
Digestive biscuit × 1	2		10
Fresh fruit × 1	2		10
Lunch			
2 wholemeal rolls	8		40
Thin spread polyunsat. margarine		10	
Lean meat 56 g	14	10	
Salad			
Low fat plain yoghurt × 1	6	1.0	10
Fresh fruit × 1	2		10
Mid-afternoon			
Tea with skimmed milk	1.0		1.5
Digestive biscuit × 2	4.0		20
Dinner			
Lean meat 84 g	21	15	
Potatoes 3 small	6		30
Vegetables			
Fresh fruit × 1	2		10
Ice cream × 1	2	4	10
Supper			
1 glass skimmed milk 200 ml	6	1.0	10
Wholemeal bread × 2	4		20
Thin spread polyunsat. margarine		10	
	95	62	233 g
Total 1870	380	558	932 kcal
	20	30	50 %
REAL			
Breakfast			
Branflakes 2 tbsp	2		10
Milk 200 ml	6	10	10
Toast 1 slice	2		10
Butter, thin spread		5	
Mid-morning			
Tea with milk	1.0	1.5	1.5
Digestive biscuit × 2		20	
Lunch			
Bread 3 slices	6		30
Butter		15	
Cheese 42 g	10	13	
Salad			

Table 7.1   (*Cont'd*)

	Protein	Fat	CHO
Fresh fruit × 1	2		10
Tea with milk	1.0	1.5	1.5
Mid-afternoon			
Tea with milk	1.0	1.5	1.5
Digestive biscuit × 1	2		10
Dinner			
Lean meat 112 g	28	20	
Potato, boiled × 2	4		20
Vegetables			
Fresh fruit × 1	2		10
Ice cream × 1	2	4	10
Supper			
1 glass milk	6	10	10
Toast 1 slice	2		10
Butter		5	
Digestive biscuit × 1	2		10
	83	87	175 g
Total 1816	333	783	700 kcal
	18	43	39 %

excluding cottage cheese), and a switch to skimmed or semi-skimmed milk with a reduction in fried food (BDA recommendations 1982).

In Asian communities it has been shown that in many groups the diet consists of a low carbohydrate and high fat content contrary to current recommendations. Chapatis (made from 85% wheat flour) are a major source of cereal fibre and ghee and cooking oil account for the high fat intake, as many eat fried food snacks. It is not always an easy task to restructure such a diet, since it is only recently that relevant and adequate diet sheets in the language of origin have been available (Peterson et al 1986).

If blood glucose control is not adequate, this will be reflected in higher concentrations shown in home blood glucose monitoring tests and a gradual rise in serial glycosylated haemoglobin levels. When diet alone is inadequate insulin treatment is started. The diet may need to be modified by redistributing the carbohydrate intake throughout the day when insulin is introduced to avoid hypoglycaemia.

Patients with an impaired glucose tolerance should eat the same diet as NIDD patients, as this may limit the degree of impairment as pregnancy advances.

Oral hypoglycaemic agents

Oral hypoglycaemic agents are not used in managing pregnant diabetic women at King's College Hospital, since it is felt that if diet alone is not sufficient to control maternal blood glucose levels insulin should be used because it is more effective.

In developing countries, where pregnant, overweight NIDD patients are common, however, oral hypoglycaemics are very useful and often more acceptable and practical than injected insulin. Coetzee & Jackson (1985–86) have proposed a regimen for the management of NIDD patients in pregnancy using an appropriately constituted calorie restricted diet and metformin or glibenclamide as necessary. Insulin is only used if the oral agents do not give satisfactory control of blood glucose levels. They report a series of 423 new diabetics diagnosed in pregnancy (i.e. 'gestational') and a further 268 known diabetics (i.e. 'established') treated in this way. The perinatal mortality rates were 14 and 70 per 1000 total births, respectively. A further 80 NIDD patients were first seen late in pregnancy and, significantly, the perinatal mortality in this group was 313/1000. Important among the observations made by these authors is the fact that side effects of oral hypoglycaemics are few and mild: they were not found to be teratogenic and starvation ketosis was not observed. Neonatal hypoglycaemia was avoided by resorting to intravenous insulin during labour. This latter step is important, since some of the oral hypoglycaemics, especially the longer-acting chlorpropamide preparation, do cross the placental barrier and exacerbate neonatal hypoglycaemia. If used they should, if possible, be discontinued 48 hours prior to delivery. The work of Coetzee & Jackson deserves special mention because of its relevance to NIDD management whenever insulin cannot be used. They have found, as have many others, in managing diabetic pregnancy that the lessons learned by the patients about diet and strict control of glucose levels help them manage their diabetes better after the pregnancy is over.

Established insulin-dependent diabetes patients

The majority of these diabetics require insulin injections at least twice daily. The most common regime uses mixtures of short-acting and medium-acting insulin mixed in the syringe and given

30 minutes before the main morning and evening meals. The actual proportion and amounts of each type of insulin are determined by gradual adjustment and by examining blood glucose profiles measured either by the patients themselves or by attendance at hospital for 12–24 hours. The aim is to achieve preprandial blood glucose levels of less than 6 mmol/l. Unacceptable swings of blood glucose often cause hypoglycaemia during the middle of the night and hyperglycaemia before breakfast. The best way to improve this twice-daily double-mixed regieme is to split the evening dose into two parts, giving the soluble insulin alone before the main evening meal and the medium-acting insulin before the bed-time snack. Greatly improved blood glucose profiles are obtained in this way (Peacock et al 1979). Alternatively before bedtime a daily dose of a medium-acting insulin supplemented by intermittent injections of short-acting insulin using a special syringe (Novopen), can be given before meals as indicated by blood glucose levels. A blood glucose level of at least 7 mmol/l is recommended before the bedtime snack if nocturnal 'hypos' are to be avoided.

Continuous subcutaneous insulin infusion (CSII)

This technique can achieve even better control than conventional insulin regimes in some patients, although during pregnancy itself it is not necessarily an advantage over the intermittent subcutaneous regime described above. It is unsuitable for emotionally labile women, whose difficulties with diabetic control are more likely to be from their personal problems rather than an intrinsic problem arising from the diabetes itself. The exact method of using CSII is described in detail by Potter et al (1981).

Starting insulin during pregnancy

In rare instances, acute insulin-dependent diabetes develops during pregnancy. Insulin treatment is then started either by using the double-mix regime or by starting with soluble insulin two or three times daily before adding the medium-acting insulin. Other patients who come to need insulin during pregnancy are the NIDD patients in whom diet alone has failed to produce adequate control. In these patients it is often sufficient to use a single dose of medium-acting insulin, starting with approximately 10 units daily. This dose can be increased, a soluble insulin added or, if need be, it can be converted into the twice-daily regime. Diabetic control after pregnancy is usually achieved with the original regime, whether diet alone or diet accompanied by an oral hypoglycaemic agent.

The insulins

Details of the commonly used insulins are shown in Table 7.2. There are no advantages to one particular type of insulin compared with any others and all are now 'purified' and at a single strength of 100 units/ml. (There has been a trend towards using porcine and 'human' insulin preparations, but there are no special advantages to the patient and no indication for changing patients from an established insulin regime using one species of insulin to another species.) Instances of insulin allergy or resistance are extremely rare.

Table 7.2 Commonly used insulins

Short-acting insulins	Intermediate-acting insulins	Long-acting insulins
		Lentard
Velosulin	Insulatard	
Humulin S	Protaphane Humulin I	Humulin Zinc
Human Actrapid	Human Monotard	
Human Velosulin	Human Insulatard	Human Ultratard

Patients should be instructed on the importance of careful timing of insulin injections before meals (30 minutes) and should be reminded of the correct injection technique and the need to rotate the site of injection from day to day.

Preconception control (see chapter 10)

Before planned pregnancies, optimal control is desirable. This is achieved using standard insulin regimes twice or three times daily. CSII can be considered where personality is appropriate and if poor diabetic control was previously responsible for fetal abnormality or loss. Patients are advised to maintain as far as possible blood glucose readings between 5 and 10 mmol/l and a glycosylated haemoglobin below 10%. Since high standards may be difficult to maintain, especially if conception is delayed, it is important not to pursue patients too relentlessly towards these goals, and cause excessive anxiety which so easily occurs in this situation.

First trimester

The need for optimal diabetic control during the first trimester has already been emphasized. Special measures are not needed but good control may be difficult to achieve. Hypoglycaemia at this stage is common, especially when the insulin dose is inappropriately increased and it is probably in part due to anorexia resulting from nausea. Although the insulin requirement increases later in pregnancy, it does not usually do so in the first trimester.

Second and third trimesters

The active cooperation of pregnant women is one factor responsible for the remarkable degree of control which is generally achieved during diabetic pregnancy without serious hypoglycaemia, but unknown physiological factors may make this easier. Diurnal and nocturnal swings of blood glucose are considerably smaller during this stage of pregnancy. Such swings, if they do occur, tend to cause hyperglycaemia after breakfast with hypoglycaemia by noon or at night. When this occurs, considerable improvement is obtained by use of the three-times-daily regime as described above. Pre-prandial blood glucose levels can usually, though not always, be maintained below 6 mmol/l. The insulin dose increases steadily through the pregnancy, especially after the 28th week. Most patients learn how to make their own adjustments to the insulin dose to maintain their control between visits to hospital. The increase in insulin requirements varies considerably, from a negligible amount to two or three times normal. Sometimes there is a small decrease in the last few weeks which is not itself an ominous feature, although if intrauterine death occurs there is a rapid decrease in insulin requirement. The need for high insulin dosage which may be reached at the end of pregnancy ceases abruptly at the time of delivery and·it is very important to reduce the dose to its pre-pregnancy level immediately after delivery, otherwise profound hypoglycaemia will develop. A careful explanation of the need for the changes in insulin dosage should be given to the pregnant diabetic, who may otherwise become anxious about the considerable increase in her total insulin dosage.

Measurement of HbA_1 throughout pregnancy is a valuable additional guide to the control which is attained (see Ch. 4). HbA_1 almost always decreases through pregnancy. The aim is to achieve normal HbA_1 levels. It is a disappointment that HbA_1 usually rises post partum.

The management of diabetes in labour is considered in Chapter 12.

REFERENCES

British Diabetic Association 1982 Dietary recommendations for diabetics for the 1980s—A policy statement by the BDA. Human Nutrition. Applied Nutrition 36A: 378-394
Coetzee E J, Jackson W P 1985–86 The management of non-insulin-dependent diabetes during pregnancy. Diabetes research and Clinical Practice 1(5): 281–287
Eastwood M A, Kay R M 1979 An hypothesis for the action of dietary fibre along the gastrointestinal tract. American Journal of Clinical Nutrition 32: 364–367
Peacock I, Hunter J C, Walford S et al 1979 Self-monitoring of blood glucose in diabetic pregnancy. British Medical Journal 2: 1333–1336
Peterson D B, Dattani J T, Baylis J M, Jepson E M 1986 Dietary practice of Asian diabetics. British Medical Journal 292: 170–171
Potter J M, Reckless J P D, Cullen D R 1981 The effect of continuous subcutaneous insulin infusion and conventional insulin regimes on 24 hour variations of blood glucose and intermediary metabolites in the third trimester of diabetic pregnancy. Diabetologia 21: 534–539

8

Obstetric management

Early pregnancy

The obstetric management of early diabetic pregnancy differs from normal in respect of an increased tendency to miscarriage and an increased risk of developing fetal abnormality. Both of these risks are reduced sharply by good diabetic control, especially if the woman has achieved good pre-conception control. Miodovnik et al (1985) showed that abortion was significantly higher in those patients with HbA_1 levels of greater than 12%. Levels of less than 12% at 8–9 weeks were associated with a favourable outcome.

Excessive nausea and vomiting and early changes in insulin requirement may make control difficult at this time. There may be a need to adjust insulin and dietary regimes to meet these difficulties although, in most cases, this will not be necessary. Early attendance at the combined diabetic antenatal clinic should ensure that diabetic control is optimal and also gives the obstetrician an opportunity to confirm that the pregnancy is proceeding normally. An early ultrasound scan establishes the maturity of the pregnancy and the size of the embryo, as well as detecting early failure of embryonic development (blighted ovum) or growth abnormality.

The combined diabetic antenatal clinic

Essential to good management of diabetic pregnancy is the combined diabetic antenatal clinic. It is also essential that diabetic physician and obstetrician work together in the same clinic, seeing the pregnant woman together. In this way both physician and obstetrician are aware of each other's problems. Free communication between the doctors involved and the patient herself greatly increases understanding and ensures the best possible patient cooperation. Diabetic women are generally well aware of the dangers of their disease in pregnancy and are well motivated to do all they can to ensure a successful outcome. The knowledge that the obstetrician and physician are working together to help them is a great encouragement. It gives them a feeling of security to know that there is a single clinic to which they can come or telephone any time during the pregnancy if they are in need of advice. Separate antenatal and diabetic clinics do not function nearly so efficiently, and cooperation between all parties concerned is more difficult: in addition, if the times at which the clinics are held differ, the patient may be involved in extra visits to the hospital.

It is usually easier for the obstetrician to go to the diabetic out-patient department for the combined clinic because of easy access to blood glucose and other necessary diabetic investigations. If this is not possible, the diabetic physician and his team should be persuaded to venture into the antenatal clinic at a set time each week. Exact arrangements for each hospital will differ, but the essential point is that there must be a combined clinic. Any hospital which is unable to achieve a combined clinic, and this may be difficult, should consider referring its pregnant diabetic patients to the nearest hospital that does.

Experience in the management of diabetic pregnancy is usually limited in the average district general hospital, so the care of such patients is best concentrated in the hands of one obstetrician and one diabetic physician. Complicated cases or patients with bad past obstetric histories are often best dealt with in a specialized centre with a wider experience of the problem. In the South East Metropolitan Region of England the average prevalence of established diabetes complicating pregnancy is approximately 1 in 500, so that a hospital delivering 2500 within a year will see only five cases per annum. Specialized diabetic antenatal clinics will see 30–50 cases annually and have the opportunity to develop special expertise in their management.

The importance of having an intensive special care baby unit in any hospital delivering diabetic women cannot be overemphasized. Here again, paediatric neonatal expertise born of experience of managing the infant of a diabetic mother in numbers is invaluable and in late pregnancy the neonatal paediatrician will often be consulted over the timing of the delivery.

Routine antenatal care

In the context of the combined diabetic antenatal clinic, the routine obstetric antenatal care of the pregnant patient does not differ greatly from that of the non-diabetic. A central role is played by diagnostic ultrasound, but this must not be allowed to obscure routine clinical observation of the patient as the pregnancy progresses. General and local abdominal examinations are important, the former giving an indication of general wellbeing and the latter in determining size and presentation of the fetus as well as giving an indication of hydramnios. Oedema of the legs is very common in late diabetic pregnancy, especially in the presence of hydramnios and a macrosomic fetus. It can usually be ignored unless accompanied by other signs of pre-eclampsia.

Pre-eclampsia and diabetic pregnancy

Pre-eclampsia, often severe, was a common occurrence in diabetic pregnancy and was equal in importance to birth trauma in causing 'obstetric' perinatal death at King's in the 1951–70 series. More recently, however, it has become much less common and there were no perinatal deaths due to pre-eclampsia at King's during the 15-year series 1971–85. Pre-eclampsia is, nevertheless, more frequent in diabetic pregnancy than in non-diabetic pregnancy. It is not clear why this should be, but it has been shown (Broughton Pipkin et al 1982) that in diabetic pregnancy the plasma renin and aldosterone concentrations are higher than in non-diabetic pregnancy and the plasma renin substrate is lower. Plasma angiotensin II showed a strong inverse relationship with serum sodium and was directly proportional to blood glucose concentration. These differences from normal, especially the tendency to higher concentrations of plasma angiotensin II, may contribute to the raised incidence of hypertension in diabetic pregnancy and explain why good control leads to a lower incidence. In the UK diabetic survey (Brudenell 1982) there was an overall incidence of pre-eclampsia of 14.4% in established diabetics and 11.6% in gestational diabetics. There was, however, no increase in perinatal mortality in those diabetic pregnancies complicated by pre-eclampsia. Thus although pre-eclampsia remains a more common occurrence in diabetic than in non-diabetic pregnancy, it does not present a particular problem in antenatal care, being detected and managed as in non-diabetic pregnancy. It is widely assumed that better diabetic control has been responsible for the falling incidence of pre-eclampsia in diabetic pregnancy and it is more likely to complicate badly controlled diabetic pregnancy. Against this must be set the general diminution of pre-eclampsia, particularly severe pre-eclampsia, that has occurred particularly in the UK over the past 2 decades.

Hydramnios in diabetic pregnancy

Hydramnios is a common feature of diabetic pregnancy, complicating 25% of pregnancies occurring in established diabetics and 13.4% of gestational diabetics in the UK diabetic survey (Brudenell 1982). The finding of hydramnios may be the first indication of gestational diabetes and when it occurs it may be responsible for preterm labour. However, the severe acute hydramnios which was responsible for four perinatal deaths at King's in the 1951–70 series has not been seen in the last 15 years. The development of hydramnios during the course of a diabetic pregnancy is an indication to look closely at the level of diabetic control that the patient is achieving, since hydramnios is more likely to occur in the badly controlled patient. The hypothesis that the hydramnios is due, at least in part, to fetal polyuria secondary to fetal hyperglycaemia is supported by the observation of fetal bladder enlargement in diabetic pregnancy (Hobbins et al 1983). As with many features of diabetic pregnancy, there seems to be a great deal of individual variation: hydramnios may feature in a well-controlled patient and be absent in one who is less well controlled. Patients who seem to be developing hydramnios quickly, i.e. over a period of 2–3 weeks in the third trimester, should be admitted to hospital for more closely supervised diabetic control and extra rest. This combination of treatment often seems to halt the progress of developing hydramnios and postpone the onset of preterm labour which otherwise may complicate it.

Frequency of antenatal visits

The frequency with which the pregnant diabetic woman attends the combined clinic will normally be determined by the diabetic physician in the first 28 weeks of the pregnancy. During this time, if diabetic control is good, fortnightly visits are adequate in many cases. More frequent visits will be needed in the latter part of the pregnancy, the exact timing depending on obstetric progress and the need for continuing strict diabetic control. Two-weekly or once-weekly visits may be required at any stage of the pregnancy, but should be avoided unless they are really necessary. The pregnant diabetic women has a good deal to cope with and too frequent visits to the clinic are an unnecessary addition to her burden. The most important point about this aspect of antenatal care is to be flexible and to plan each patient's clinic visits according to her needs. It is, of course, essential that the patient herself should feel free to contact or visit the clinic at any time during the pregnancy if she feels at all anxious about her diabetic control or the progress of the pregnancy.

The use of ultrasound in diabetic pregnancy (Table 8.1)

The advent of diagnostic ultrasound has made an important impact on the management of diabetic pregnancy.

Table 8.1 Diagnostic ultrasound scanning in diabetic pregnancy

Before 12 weeks	At 18–20 weeks	From 24 weeks onwards
Maturity	Most major congenital abnormalities including cardiac abnormality	Regular scans indicate fetal growth and detect developing macrosomia
Embryo growth and development (blighted ovum)	Amniocentesis in some cases	Liquor volume to detect hydramnios OR oligohydramnios
Multiple pregnancy	Confirmation of maturity	Placental size and position
Gross congenital abnormality		Placental and fetal blood flow
Ultrasound directed chorion villus biopsy		Fetal activity

Before 12 weeks

As indicated above, a scan in early pregnancy is valuable as a means of establishing both maturity and the wellbeing of the embryo, as well as detecting gross abnormality. Pedersen & Mølsted-Pedersen (1979) found that the crown–rump lengths in diabetic pregnancy were, on average, 5.4 days smaller than those in non-diabetic pregnancy of the same menstrual age. This surprising finding has been confirmed by other observers (Pedersen et al, in further studies, 1984, 1985) but was disputed by Little et al (1979) and Steel (1988). Harper and Morrow (1988) point out the difficulties in proving early growth delay because of the occurrence of delayed ovulation resulting in late conception. Pedersen suggests on the basis of HbA_{1c} measurements in 40 diabetic women that early fetal growth delay may result from poor diabetic control. It is always wise to confirm maturity at a later stage in the pregnancy by biparietal diameter and femur length measurements. Multiple pregnancy and gross congenital abnormality may also be detected at the early pregnancy scan, although the latter will be looked for again at 18 weeks. Ultrasound directed chorion villus biopsy does not have a special part to play in diabetic antenatal care, but may be preferred as a means for screening for Down's syndrome in diabetic women over the age of 35.

18–20 weeks

A detailed fetal anomaly scan is an essential part of the antenatal care of all pregnant diabetics. This scan should be performed by an ultrasonographer skilled and experienced in the detection of all forms of fetal anomaly, including cardiac anomaly. This is particularly important in those women whose diabetic control in the first trimester, as indicated by blood glucose levels (if available) or an HbA_1 estimation of greater than 12%, has been bad (see p. 23). Amniocentesis is indicated in women of 35 years of age or over, as a screening test for Down's syndrome, and is also helpful if there is a suspicion of neural tube defect. Maternal serum alpha-fetoprotein (AFP) levels measured between 12 and 24 weeks' gestation are 60% of the levels found in non-diabetic pregnancy (Wald et al 1979). The interpretation of AFP levels depends upon a knowledge of the gestational age of the pregnancy, since the levels rise progressively in the second trimester with increasing gestation. Accurate dating of the pregnancy using both ultrasound data and the menstrual history should eliminate this source of error in interpreting AFP levels in diabetic women. Milunsky et al (1982) recommend that the upper limit cut-off level of AFP levels for diabetic women should be 2.0 or 2.5 times median on a normal pregnancy curve, but at a point equivalent to 2 weeks earlier. There is no known cause for the lower level of maternal serum AFP in diabetic women, although the finding is most marked when the diabetes is badly controlled (Szabo et al 1986). This investigation may prove a worthwhile addition to routine diabetic antenatal care, although at the present time it offers no obvious clinical advantage. In practice, neural tube defects and associated meningomyelocoeles are almost invariably detected by an experienced ultrasonographer, but an appropriate elevation in the amniotic alphafetoprotein level confirms the diagnosis. Fetal maturity can be confirmed at this examination by measuring the biparietal diameter of the fetal head and the length of the femur. An estimate of maturity based on these two measurements will give a better prediction of expected date of delivery than the menstrual history (Campbell & Wilkin 1975). This is important, as the menstrual cycle is often irregular in diabetic women.

From 24 weeks onwards

One of the major remaining problems associated with diabetic pregnancy is the development of diabetic fetal macrosomia. This may occur even though the maternal diabetes is impeccably controlled (see Ch. 9). Evidence of fetal macrosomia can be obtained by serial measurements of the fetal abdominal and head circumferences, starting at 24 weeks and continuing at 2-weekly intervals until delivery. Developing macrosomia is evident by 32 or 34 weeks, and is an indication that the maternal diabetes may be affecting fetal growth. As noted in Chapter 13, Flynn et al (1986) have demonstrated an increased velocity of growth in macrosomic babies at an earlier stage in pregnancy. Macrosomia may, of course, occur in the absence of maternal diabetes, but it is wise to assume that macrosomia developing in a pregnant diabetic woman is due to the maternal diabetes and act accordingly. If the maternal diabetes is not well controlled urgent steps must be taken to improve control. Once macrosomia has started to develop it usually continues to do so, regardless of any such improvements. The important practical advantage gained by ultrasound detection of macrosomia is that the obstetrician is warned of possible intrauterine fetal anoxia and dystocia and can plan the timing and mode of delivery.

Macrosomia is accompanied by an increase in placental size. If the thickness of the placenta as measured at right angles to its long axis exceeds 5 cm a large placenta should be suspected. However, if hydramnios is present the placenta may become stretched out over an expanded uterus and the increased size therefore not evident. A homogeneous appearance of the placental substance is rarely seen after 30 weeks in normal pregnancy, but is sometimes seen in diabetic women at this time. Hydramnios, as noted above, is more common in diabetic pregnancy and can be visualized on ultrasound scanning. The fetal bladder often appears unduly large (Hobbins et al 1983), probably as a result of fetal polyuria secondary to poor diabetic control. Occasionally the finding of a large fetal bladder has been the means of diagnosing gestational diabetes. Oligohydramnios may also be seen complicating intrauterine growth retardation in a diabetic pregnancy. It is usually associated with vascular complications in the mother, especially diabetic nephropathy and chronic hypertension.

Fetal movements in utero are readily observed during ultrasound scanning and form part of the biophysical profile commonly used to evaluate fetal wellbeing. Maternal blood glucose levels within the normoglycaemic range (3.3–7.8 mmol/l) do not affect fetal movements, nor does hyperglycaemia (>7.8 mmol/l). Maternal blood glucose levels of less than 3.3 mmol/l are accompanied by a significant increase in fetal activity (Holden et al 1984). Fetal movement patterns vary considerably in normal pregnancy, but a reduction in movement persisting for 12 hours (Sadowsky & Polishnik 1977) calls for urgent evaluatlon of the fetal condition, taking all other factors, growth pattern, fetal ECG, liquor volume, etc. into consideration. Fetal breathing movements have attracted particular attention, and there is strong evidence that they cease when the fetus is hypoxic (Roberts et al 1979). However, in a group of 25 diabetic pregnancies studied at King's College Hospital (Roberts et al 1980) fetal respiratory and trunk movements were significantly higher than in non-diabetics. Marked reductions in fetal trunk activity correlated with abnormal stress tests and fetal distress in labour, while reductions in fetal respiratory movements did not. In practice, however, reduction of fetal movements generally or trunk movements in particular gives a rather late warning of fetal distress in utero, and since these observations are time consuming they are of little help in assessing fetal wellbeing in diabetic pregnancy generally.

Blood flow studies

Wave forms from the fetal and maternal side of the placental circulation can readily be measured using a duplexed pulsed Doppler system. Quantitative measurement of blood flow may be subject to large errors, but useful information is gained by a study of the flow velocity wave forms (Campbell et al 1984). Absent end diastolic frequencies in the fetal aorta or impaired flow through the arcuate arteries on the maternal side of the placenta are found in association with intrauterine growth retardation. Studies at King's College Hospital indicate that uteroplacental blood flow in diabetic pregnancy is normal: there is an increase in fetal aortic blood flow velocity related to the degree of developing macrosomia. The exact value of this investigation in diabetic pregnancy, except when complicated by intrauterine growth retardation, remains to be seen. It is easily performed, however, and should now be added to the routine investigation of a diabetic fetus in late pregnancy as an additional measurement of fetal wellbeing.

Cordocentesis in diabetic pregnancy

The proposition that fetal hypoxia is the cause of late intrauterine fetal death in diabetic pregnancy, made by Brudenell 1987 and more fully reported by Bradley et al (1988), was based on the findings of a cordocentesis study carried out at King's College Hospital. The technique of cordocentesis allows the antenatal sampling of pure fetal blood taken from the umbilical cord through a needle introduced under ultrasound control. In the series of 16 patients examined in the study, the PO_2 was found to be lower than the mean in the majority of cases, especially toward the end of pregnancy. Some fetuses were also found to be relatively hypoxic as early as 20 weeks. In addition to the changes in PO_2, the PCO_2 was found to be elevated, although there was no change in the pH from normal values. Although cordocentesis seems unlikely to become a routine procedure in the antenatal monitoring of fetal wellbeing in diabetic pregnancy, its value in selected cases was illustrated in a case report (Bradley et al 1988) of an insulin-dependent diabetic who was found on routine Doppler studies to have a high resistance index in the utero-placental circulation. At this time, cordocentesis revealed a PO_2 of 36.8 mmHg and a pH of 7.33. Fetal growth was normal and the diabetic control good. At 29 weeks the fetal blood flows in both utero-placental and umbilical cord circulation were abnormal and a further cordocentesis at this time confirmed that the fetus had become hypoxic—PO_2 25.3 mmHg but not acidotic, pH 7.35. As other fetal parameters were normal, the pregnancy was allowed to continue but at 31 weeks the fetal heart trace showed deep decelerations. The cord PO_2 at this time had fallen to 24.4 mmHg and the pH to 7.31. The baby was delivered by caesarean section with a pH of 7.20 and an Apgar score of 3 at 1 minute. It subsequently recovered and was normal on discharge home at 22 days. It is likely that had this pregnancy been allowed to continue the baby would have been at serious risk of intra-uterine death from anoxia.

Late pregnancy—admission to hospital

In well-controlled, uncomplicated diabetic pregnancy antenatal care can follow a normal pattern up to full term. If there is any particular cause for concern in the last 6 weeks of pregnancy (e.g. difficulty in diabetic control, developing hydramnios or pre-eclampsia) patients should be admitted to hospital so that diabetic control can be closely supervised and fetal wellbeing monitored. Patients whose serial ultrasound scans show developing fetal macrosomia come into this category, since the excessive growth of the fetus is a clear indication that it is being affected by the maternal diabetes, however well controlled this may be. Whilst it has been shown that diabetic control can be better at home than in hospital (Stubbs et al 1980), this only applies to well-motivated patients making regular checks of their blood glucose levels. Less intelligent or less well-motivated patients are likely to be better controlled in hospital. Good control is, of course, especially important in the last few weeks of pregnancy when the other complications may arise. Hospital in-patient supervision does offer the best chance of optimal obstetric and diabetic care. It may be argued that this is an unnecessarily cautious approach, but the last few weeks of diabetic pregnancy see the culmination of a great deal of effort on the part of the patient and the diabetic/obstetric team which is totally wasted if there is a perinatal death. For this reason, a cautious approach including hospital admission seems justified.

Monitoring of fetal wellbeing in late diabetic pregnancy

Because of the occurrence of 'unexplained' late intrauterine fetal death in diabetic pregnancy, considerable attention has been focused on monitoring fetal wellbeing at this time. In practice, this classic complication is only rarely seen in the well-controlled diabetic: when it does occur it seems to do so without prior warning and so far no satisfactory test has been discovered that will predict it. Fetal hypoxia may occur in diabetic as in non-diabetic pregnancy as the result of 'placental insufficiency'. It is then most often a complication of maternal hypertension which, as noted above, not infrequently complicates diabetic pregnancy. As indicated in Chapter 11, there is now good evidence that fetal hypoxia also occurs in diabetic pregnancy when the placenta and fetus appear to be of normal or greater than normal size. The fact that the diabetic fetus may be hypoxic in late pregnancy explains why fetal distress in labour is more common in diabetic pregnancy, especially as hyperglycaemia exaggerates the effect of even mild anoxia (Shelley et al 1975). The late fetal deaths tend to occur in badly-controlled diabetics (as evidenced by fetal pancreatic beta cell hypertrophy and hyperplasia) (Cardell 1953). The fetus is usually macrosomic.

In a well-controlled normotensive diabetic with normal fetal growth, it is probably true that no tests for fetal wellbeing are required. When fetal growth is excessive or the mother hypertensive or badly controlled the fetus is at greater risk and tests of fetal wellbeing are then of particular value. In practice, all diabetic women in late pregnancy are customarily subjected to fetal monitoring to a greater or lesser extent.

Biochemical tests

Serial estimations of maternal urinary or serum oestriol levels were widely used and are still advocated by some authors. Goh et al (1982) found that serial measurements of plasma oestriol concentrations gave a detection rate of approximately 85% for both normal and abnormal fetal outcomes in 96 diabetic and 192 normal pregnancies. There were 15% false negative and 16% false positive results. Jorge et al (1981) combined serial oestriol estimations with biophysical tests and found that an abnormal oestriol value preceded abnormal heart rate testing in 8 out of 10 patients. Their conclusion, however, was that their combined method of testing of fetal wellbeing was most helpful in determining when not to intervene, so allowing safe prolongation of pregnancy. Dooley et al (1984) found that in only 2 out of 21 patients showing a 40% oestriol drop was there fetal distress indicated by non-stress cardiotocography. Chronic low levels of oestriol were related to smaller placentas but not fetal jeopardy. Freinkel et al (1985), on the basis of the findings of Dooley, have abandoned routine estimations of oestriol levels in favour of biophysical testing. At King's College Hospital serial urinary oestriol output levels were measured routinely in all patients in late pregnancy, but the considerable within-patient and patient-to-patient variation in levels made interpretation of results difficult. Only in relatively rare incidences of fetal intra-uterine growth retardation complicating diabetic pregnancies were oestriol levels found to be of value. The same general conclusions apply to serial measurements of serum levels of human placental lactogen, which were also used at King's (Ursell et al 1973). Biochemical tests have been completely superceded by biophysical tests in the past 5 years and there has, so far, been no reason to regret this change.

Biophysical testing

Biophysical tests provide a more direct assessment of fetal wellbeing than biochemical tests and for this reason have grown in popularity in recent times. However, their limitations in respect of the detection of unexplained late intrauterine fetal death in diabetic pregnancy are probably the same. They do, however, provide immediate evidence of intrauterine fetal anoxia due to placental insufficiency and so are of particular value in cases of intrauterine fetal growth retardation, hypertension and pre-eclampsia complicating diabetic pregnancy. Their value in uncomplicated late diabetic pregnancy remains to be proven. At present they are widely applied as a precautionary measure, especially when the pregnancy is being allowed to proceed to full term.

Fetal movement recording

Fetal movements cease some variable time before fetal death occurs. The assessment of fetal activity by the patient is a simple and effective way of detecting developing fetal hypoxia, but has not proved to be of particular value in uncomplicated diabetic pregnancy. The kick count described by Pearson & Weaver (1976) is a practical way of using this approach, the patient noting the time taken from 9 a.m. for the fetus to make ten definite movements. This should be achieved in under 12 hours. At King's College Hospital those diabetic patients who are admitted to hospital in late pregnancy are currently asked to do a daily kick count. Although no definite clinical advantage has been gained from these observations, their psychological value to the patients should not be underrated.

Antenatal fetal heart monitoring (cardiotocography)

Most recent papers on the management of diabetic pregnancy advocate the use of this test of fetal wellbeing in late pregnancy (Golde et al 1984, Freinkel et al 1985, Gillmer 1985, Landon & Gabbe 1985, Miller & Horger 1985). Both oxytocin stress and non-stress tests have been used, although the latter seems the more popular and is the one currently employed at King's College Hospital. As with other methods of fetal monitoring, the main application of the non-stress test is to cases of suspected fetal anoxia and abnormal tests are rarely seen in uncomplicated diabetic pregnancy. Olufsson et al (1986) reported that only 3.7% of 2672 non-stress tests in 99 diabetic pregnancies were pathological. They found that a normal test performed within 2 days of delivery predicted an Apgar score of greater than 7 at 1 minute in 92% and at 5 and 10 minutes in 99%. When complications occur, especially in maternal hypertension, hydramnios, developing fetal macrosomia or intrauterine fetal growth retardation the patient is admitted to hospital and daily fetal heart monitoring is carried out. It is most often useful in encouraging the obstetrician that there is no immediate need to interfere with the pregnancy. A non-reactive or otherwise abnormal test indicates immediate and careful assessment of the situation. A full fetal biophysical profile is then performed, including fetal and maternal blood flow measurements. If there is any doubt about fetal wellbeing, immediate induction of labour or delivery by caesarean section is called for. One factor that needs to be taken into account in assessing fetal heart traces in diabetics is the effect of maternal hypoglycaemia. Stangenberg et al (1983) and Langer and Cohens (1984) noted a decrease in fetal heart rate and variability during episodes of maternal hypoglycaemia. The fetal heart trace returned to normal when the maternal blood glucose was raised to normal levels.

The biophysical profile

The fetal biophysical profile is a combination of fetal attributes designed to improve the accuracy of the diagnosis of fetal anoxia. In addition to non-stress cardiotocography the fetus is observed using a real time ultrasound scanner and observations are made on fetal breathing movements, fetal body movements, fetal tone and amniotic fluid volume. By using this test, Manning (1982) reduced the false negative rate in the diagnosis of fetal hypoxia to less than 1 in 1000 in 3100 non-diabetic pregnancies. For the diabetic fetus at risk, the biophysical profile is helpful in providing reassurance to the clinician that he can continue with a conservative policy in regard to delivery if it is appropriate on clinical criteria to do so. It may also indicate the need for early delivery in complicated diabetic pregnancy. In the future cordocentesis may be added to the biophysical profile and used in selected cases to confirm fetal hypoxia and assess its severity.

Conclusions

The outcome of a diabetic pregnancy rests primarily on the quality of antenatal care provided both by the diabetic physician and the obstetrician, working closely together as a combined team. The best possible care will, however, fail if the patient is unable or unwilling to cooperate: her understanding of the problems her pregnancy poses is therefore essential. Given this basis, the great majority of diabetic pregnancies will end successfully. Diagnostic ultrasound has greatly improved the ability of the obstetrician to monitor fetal wellbeing throughout the pregnancy and to detect any adverse effects which the maternal diabetes, even when well controlled, may have on it.

REFERENCES

Broughton Pipkin F, Hunter J C, Oats J J N, O'Brien P M S 1982 The renin angiotensin system in normal and diabetic pregnancy. In: Sammour M B, Symonds E M, Zuspan F P, El Tomi N (eds) Pregnancy hypertension. Ain Sham University Press, pp 185–192

Bradley P J, Nicolaides K H, Brudenell J M, Campbell S 1988 Early diagnosis of fetal hypoxia in a diabetic pregnancy. British Medical Journal 296: 94–95

Brudenell M 1982 Obstetric complications in the antenatal period in diabetic pregnancy. Results of UK Diabetic Pregnancy Survey, Beard R W, Lowy C, RCOG Scientific Meeting 1982

Brudenell J M 1987 Fletcher Shaw Lecture, Royal College of Obstetricians and Gynaecologists

Campbell S, Wilkin D 1975 Ultrasonic meausurement of fetal abdominal circumference in the estimation of fetal weight. British Journal of Obstetrics and Gynaecology 82: 689–697

Campbell S, Hernandez C J, Cohen-Overbeck T A, Pearce J M F 1984 Assessment of feto-placental and utero-placental blood flow using duplex pulsed Doppler ultrasound in complicated pregnancy. Journal of Perinatal Medicine 12: 262–265

Cardell B S 1953 Hypertrophy and hyperplasia of the pancreatic islets in newborn infants. Journal of Pathology and Bacteriology 2: 335–346

Dooley S L, Depp R, Socol M L, Tamura R K, Vaisrab N 1984 Urinary oestriols in diabetic pregnancy: a reappraisal. Obstetrics and Gynecology 64 (4): 469–475

Flynn M D, Doddridge M, Watkins P, Brudenell M 1986 Presentation to the British Diabetic Association Meeting

Freinkel N, Dooley S L, Metzger B E 1985 Care of the pregnant woman with insulin-dependent diabetes mellitus. New England Journal of Medicine 313 (2): 96–101

Gillmer M 1985 Obstetric management of diabetes. Practical Diabetes 2 (6): 4–5

Goh H H, Lim L S, Wong P C, Ratnam S S 1982 Plasma oestriol in pregnancies complicated by diabetes mellitus. Australian Journal of Experimental Biological Medical Science 60 (5): 529–540

Golde S H, Montoro M, Good- Anderson B et al 1984 The role of non-stress tests, fetal biophysical profile and contraction stress tests in the out- patient management of insulin requiring diabetic pregnancies. American Journal of Obstetrics and Gynecology 148 (3): 269–273

Harper M A, Morrow R J 1988 Early growth delay in diabetic pregnancy. British Medical Journal 296: 1005–1006

Hobbins J C, Winsberg F, Berkowitz R L 1983 In: Ultrasonography in obstetrics and gynaecology, 2nd edn. Wilkins & Wilkins, Baltimore/London, p. 78

Holden K P, Jovanovic L, Druzen M L, Peterson C M 1984 Increased fetal activity with low maternal blood glucose levels in pregnancies complicated by diabetes. American Journal of Perinatology I (2): 161–164

Jorge C S, Artal R, Paul R H et al 1981 Anterpartum fetal surveillance in diabetic pregnant patients. American Journal of Obstetrics and Gynecology 141 (6): 641–645

Landon M B, Gabbe S 1985 Antepartum fetal surveillance in gestational diabetes mellitus. Diabetes 34 (2): 50–54

Langer O, Cohen W R 1984 Persistent fetal bradycardia during maternal hypoglycaemia. American Journal of Obstetrics and Gynecology 149 (6): 688–690

Little D J, Stubbs S M, Brudenell M et al 1979 Early growth retardation in diabetic pregnancy. British Medical Journal 282: 488

Manning F A 1982 Antepartum determination of fetal health. Clinics in Perinatology 9: 285–287

Miller J M Jnr, Horger E O 1985 Antepartum heart rate testing in diabetic pregnancy. Journal of Reproductive Medicine 30 (7): 515–518

Milunsky A, Alpert E, Kitzmiller J L, Donna Younger R 1982 The importance of serum alpha-fetoprotein screening in diabetic pregnant women. American Journal of Obstetrics and Gynecology 142: 1030–1032

Miodovnik M, Skillman C, Holroyd J C, Butler J B, Wendel J S, Sidiqi T A 1985 Elevated maternal glycohaemoglobin in early pregnancy and spontaneous abortion among insulin dependent diabetic women. American Journal of Obstetrics and Gynecology 153 (4): 439–442

Olufsson P, Sjoberg N O, Solum T 1986 Fetal surveillance in diabetic pregnancy. Predictive value of the non-stress test. Acta Obstetrica et Gynecologica Scandinavia 65: 241–246

Pearson J F, Weaver J B 1976 Fetal activity and fetal well being—an evaluation. British Medical Journal 1: 1305–1307

Pedersen J F, Mølsted-Pedersen L 1979 Early fetal growth retardation in diabetic pregnancy. British Medical Journal 1: 18–19

Pedersen J F, Mølsted Pedersen L, Mortenson H B 1984 Fetal growth and maternal HbA$_{1c}$ in early diabetic pregnancy. Obstetrics and Gynecology 84, 64 (3): 351–352

Pedersen J F, Mølsted-Pedersen L 1985 The possibility of an early growth delay in White's class A diabetic pregnancy. Diabetes 34 (2) 47–49

Roberts A B, Little D, Cooper D, Campbell S 1979 Normal patterns of fetal activity in the third trimester. British Journal of Obstetrics and Gynaecology 86: 4–9

Roberts A B, Stubbs S M, Brudenell M et al 1980 Fetal activity in pregnancies complicated by maternal diabetes. British Journal of Obstetrics and Gynaecology 87: 485–489

Sadowsky E, Polishnik W Z 1977 Fetal movements in utero: nature, assessment, prognostic value, timing of delivery. Obstetrics and Gynecology 50: 49–55

Shelley H J, Basset J M, Milner R D G 1975 Control of carbohydrate metabolism in the fetus and newborn. British Medical Bulletin 31: 37–43

Stangenberg M, Pearson B, Strange L, Carlstrom K 1983 Insulin induced hypoglycaemia in pregnant diabetics. Maternal and fetal cardiovascular reactions. Acta Obstetrica et Gynecologica Scandinavia 62 (3): 249–252

Steel J 1988 Preconception and contraception. In : Reece E A, Constan D R (Eds) Diabetes Mellitus in Pregnancy. Churchill Livingstone p 611–614

Stubbs S M, Brudenell J M, Pyke D A, Watkins P J, Stubbs W A, Alberti K G M M 1980 Management of the pregnant diabetic: Home or hospital, with or without glucose meters. Lancet i: 1122

Szabo M, Toth T, Toth Z, Szerfert G T, Csecsa K, Veress L, Papp Z 1986 Fetal malformation and serum alpha-fetoprotein concentration of diabetic mothers. Zentralblatt fur Gynaekologie 108 (20): 1228–1236

Ursell W, Brudenell M, Chard T 1973 Placental lactogen levels in diabetic pregnancy. British Medical Journal 2: 80–82

Wald N J, Cuckle H, Boreham J, Stirrut G M, Turnbull A C 1979 Maternal Serum alpha-fetoprotein and diabetes mellitus. British Journal of Obstetrics and Gynaecology 86: 101–105

9

Delivering the infant

As diabetic pregnancy nears term, the question of delivery needs careful consideration especially in respect of timing and mode. Timing will often be taken out of the clinician's hands by the onset of preterm labour, which at King's College Hospital complicates 17% of diabetic pregnancies.

Management of preterm labour*

Faced with the diabetic woman in preterm labour the immediate decision is whether or not to try and stop the labour. As a general rule, if the pregnancy has reached 32 weeks no such attempt should be made. The same applies to spontaneous rupture of membranes unaccompanied by uterine contractions at, or after 32 weeks: in this case, however, since there is likely to be a delay before the onset of contractions a sample of liquor should, if possible, be obtained either by a vaginal collection or ultrasound directed amniocentesis, and the maturity of the fetal lungs assessed (see Ch. 8). If the fetal lungs are immature a course of dexamethasone (4 mg 8-hourly for 48 hours) or beta-methasone (12 mg daily for 2 days) should be given to accelerate lung maturation. In all cases of preterm labour a sample of liquor obtained by amniocentesis or a vaginal swab should be sent for bacteriological examination and the patient, meanwhile, started on amoxycillin to counter the risk of intrauterine infection, especially by beta haemolytic streptococci. Alternative or

---

* Preterm labour is defined as the onset of labour prior to the completion of the 37th week.

additional antibiotics can be added if indicated when the bacteriological examination results are available. Preterm labour with intact or ruptured membranes before 32 weeks should generally be stopped unless it is clear that the labour is fully established as evident by the strength and frequency of the contractions and by cervical dilatation. Each case needs to be considered on its merits, however, and the size of the fetus and the presence of additional complications, especially pre-eclampsia, need to be taken into account. Beta agonists such as salbutamol or ritodrine used to inhibit uterine contractions and corticosteroids used to accelerate lung maturation may cause hyperglycaemia and subsequent ketoacidosis and hypo-kalaemia (Leslie & Coats 1977, Thomas et al 1977). Acute pulmonary oedema has also been reported in patients given beta-mimetics and corticosteroids, particularly after prolonged or repeated administration of the beta-mimetics. It commonly occurs after delivery and abrupt withdrawal of the agent (Pearce 1985). If they are to be used special precautions must be taken:

1. An intravenous infusion of soluble insulin administered by an infusion pump is set up before corticosteroids or beta agonists are given. A rate of 16 units per hour or more is often necessary to keep blood glucose levels within the normal range of 3–6 mmol/l. Once the insulin infusion has been set up the course of dexamethasone or betamethasone can be started.
2. Salbutamol, 10 mg/l or ritodrine, 100 mg/l in normal saline is given by intravenous drip at a rate adequate to control contractions without causing undue maternal hypertension or tachycardia.
3. The blood glucose level is estimated every hour and plasma potassium every 2 hours. An intravenous 5% glucose drip may be needed to counteract hypoglycaemia, and intravenous potassium supplements up to 100 mmol/24 h to maintain normal potassium levels may need to be given.
4. The maternal pulse rate and blood pressure are taken hourly and a continuous cardiotocograph trace taken of the fetal heart. Maternal hypertension or tachycardia are managed by reducing the dose of beta agonists. Maternal sweating, nausea, vomiting and tremor may occur but are not usually severe and can usually be ignored. The risk of acute pulmonary oedema must be borne in mind.

The above regimen is continued for 48 hours. If the membranes are ruptured, no further attempts should be made to inhibit labour and delivery should be allowed to occur vaginally, or in some cases (see below) a caesarean section should be performed. If the membranes are intact and the contractions have been successfully inhibited the beta agonist infusion is slowly scaled down over the succeeding 48 hours. The insulin infusion should be continued at the appropriate rate until the beta agonist is discontinued, the dose being adjusted according to blood glucose levels. Preterm labour often recurs after successful initial inhibition and the regime may have to be reinstated. In any lull between the preterm labour 'storms', amniocentesis to obtain a liquor sample for fetal lung maturity should be performed. A mature fetal lung may encourage the obstetrician to abandon attempts to inhibit labour again. If the pregnancy proceeds, a repeat course of corticosteroids should be given at 10-day intervals after the first until 32 weeks. The management of the diabetic patient in threatened preterm labour calls for a very close supervision of the patient and her fetus by the obstetric and diabetic teams and is an occasion when the highest level of cooperation between the two teams is needed. The patient needs much reassurance in what is, for her, a very frightening situation.

Caesarean section in preterm diabetic labour

When it is clear that preterm delivery cannot be prevented caesarean section should be considered. If it seems likely that labour and vaginal delivery will be straightforward there is no indication for operation. In the presence of added complications such as severe pre-eclampsia, unstable or mal presentation or increased risk of intrauterine infection a caesarean section should be performed. Each case needs to be considered individually, but vaginal delivery is generally possible and to be preferred.

Delivery after 37 weeks

Unless complications occur which necessitate earlier delivery, diabetic pregnant patients are not nowadays delivered before 37 weeks. In the well-controlled, uncomplicated diabetic with normal fetal growth, pregnancy is allowed to proceed to 40 weeks. Once the patient has reached full term it is the present policy at King's College Hospital to induce labour or, if indicated (see below) deliver by caesarean section. Mølsted Pedersen & Kuhl (1986) feel that the increased risk of late intrauterine death still exists in late diabetic pregnancy and in general induce labour around the 38th week. Other writers (Drury 1984, 1986, Murphy et al 1984) have maintained that in such patients there is no need to intervene and that labour can be allowed to start spontaneously and proceed normally. However, it must be said that experience in the management of diabetic pregnancy that has gone beyond 40 weeks is, at present, limited. For the time being at least, therefore, the 'deliver at 40 weeks' rule for uncomplicated diabetic pregnancy is still recommended. It may be argued that with modern methods of monitoring fetal wellbeing this is an unnecessarily conservative (= intervention in this context) approach, but since monitoring of fetal wellbeing, especially in diabetic pregnancy, is still an imprecise art the known additional risks of induction of labour at 40 weeks seem less than the unknown risks of 'post maturity'.

Planned caesarean section

Every effort should be made to avoid complicated difficult or prolonged labour in diabetic women. Planned caesarean section will, therefore, be appropriate in a number of cases and will usually be performed between 38 and 40 weeks. The natural desire of all women to have a normal vaginal delivery must always be respected, but the diabetic woman is sensible of the additional hazards she may face in labour and will usually accept a carefully considered decision to deliver by caesarean section. It is wise to discuss the increased chance of having an abdominal delivery with diabetic women during the course of the pregnancy.

Indications

The indications for planned caesarian section in diabetic pregnancy are:

Previous caesarean section;
Malpresentation;
Disproportion;

Severe pre-eclampsia;
Age 35 or over;
Long history of infertility;
Diabetic complications.

Previous caesarean section

This is a common indication for caesarean section in diabetic women. Although the risk of scar rupture in labour is slight, it is not usually acceptable in the diabetic. Individual women may have a strong desire for vaginal delivery and for them a trial of scar may be appropriate. In general, however, the 'once a caesarean always a caesarean' rule should apply to diabetic pregnancy. Most diabetic women will aim to have small families, so the surgical problems of repeat operation should not be excessive. Nevertheless, any repeat caesarean operation should be performed by a skilled obstetric surgeon.

Malpresentation

Unstable or breech presentation should be delivered abdominally: once again, the slight additional risk to the fetus imposed by attempting a vaginal delivery is unacceptable.

Disproportion

The prevalence of macrosomia means that the risk of disproportion and difficult vaginal delivery is always present. Birth trauma has often featured in diabetic deliveries in earlier series (Stallone & Ziel 1974) and was a major cause of perinatal mortality at King's College Hospital in 1951–70 (see Ch. 11). When macrosomia has been detected by serial ultrasound scanning and it seems likely that dystocia will result, serious consideration must be given to a planned caesarean section. Shoulder dystocia is a particular risk for the macrosomic diabetic fetus. Acker et al (1985) found that 31% of delivered diabetic neonates weighing 4000 g or more experienced shoulder dystocia. These authors recommend planned caesarean section for the delivery of any diabetic fetus whose antenatal weight prediction is 4000 g or more. No hard and fast rules can be laid down, but a trial of labour for a suspected disproportion should be a rare event in diabetic pregnancy and if embarked upon should be short.

Pre-eclampsia

Severe pre-eclampsia is best treated by caesarean section. It may often arise as a complication of pre-existing hypertension or diabetic nephropathy. Eclampsia is fortunately rare in diabetic pregnancy, but requires a caesarean section as soon as the fits have been controlled.

Maternal age and infertility

These indications are relative and each case must be judged on its merits.

Diabetic complications

Women with moderate or severe diabetic microvasculopathy are more likely to develop obstetric complications, particularly pre-eclampsia and fetal intrauterine growth retardation. They will best be delivered by planned caesarean section.

Other indications

These include patients who have a bad past obstetric history either of a perinatal death or a difficult labour. A subsequent pregnancy imposes an extra physical and mental strain on the patient and delivery itself may present a psychological barrier which is best overcome by a planned caesarean section.

Management of planned caesarean section

Obstetric management

This is no different from that in non-diabetic pregnancy. General anaesthesia or epidural analgesia are appropriate, and the choice can usually be made by the patient herself after discussion with the obstetrician and anaesthetist concerned. If epidural analgesia is used the management of the maternal diabetes is easier, as the patient is able to take carbohydrate by mouth in the immediate postoperative period when insulin requirement falls sharply. It is generally preferable to manage the pre- and intraoperative period by intravenous glucose and insulin and in the case of section under general anaesthesia this regime is continued until the patient is able to take fluids freely by mouth.

Diabetics who are delivered by caesarean section either as a planned procedure or in labour are at increased risk of postoperative intrauterine and wound infection (Diamond et al 1986). Every care should be taken to avoid infection, and if the risk seems particularly high, prophylactic antibiotics are appropriate.

Medical management

If the operation is planned for the morning, the long-acting insulin is omitted the previous night as well as all insulin on the morning of the operation. An insulin and glucose infusion is set up as for diabetic labour. If the operation is to take place in the afternoon, the long-acting insulin is given the previous evening along with the short-acting insulin. In the morning, half of the short-acting insulin is given as usual before breakfast and the intravenous glucose and insulin infusions started 2 hours preoperatively. The aim is a blood glucose level between 4 and 6 mmol/l.

Induction of labour

The indication for induction of labour in diabetic pregnancy has changed during the past decade, reflecting the growing confidence which obstetricians have in managing the well-controlled patient. At King's College Hospital in such women the risk of late, unexplained intrauterine death up to full term has virtually disappeared and so uncomplicated diabetes per se does not now normally constitute an indication to induce labour.

Indications

The indications for induction of labour are:

Fullterm pregnancy;
Developing fetal macrosomia;
Gestational hypertension (if severe);
Pre-eclampsia;
Chronic hypertension;
Diabetic microvasculopathy.

Fullterm uncomplicated diabetes

Once the diabetic woman reaches full term it is, as indicated above, the present policy at King's College Hospital to induce labour. This policy is kept under constant review, and as experience in the outcome of diabetic pregnancy allowed to go past term increases it may be necessary to change to a less interventionist approach. The results of the present approach are satisfactory in terms of perinatal mortality and morbidity, and no change will be made until it is clear that it will not involve an increased risk for the fetus.

Developing fetal macrosomia

A fetus that is growing excessively as judged by serial ultrasound scans is clearly being affected by the maternal diabetes and becoming hyperinsulinaemic. The hyperinsulinaemic, macrosomic fetus is the one who is likely to be hypoxic and therefore at greatest risk of late intrauterine death (see Ch. 11). In such cases it seems prudent to induce labour at 38 weeks, in view of the possible risk of late intrauterine death in the remaining 2 weeks of the pregnancy. The risk of failed induction is small at this time, and by eliminating the increase in fetal size that would otherwise occur in the last 2 weeks, or more if the woman is allowed to go past term, the risk of dystocia due to disproportion is also reduced.

Pre-eclampsia

The indications for induction for pre-eclampsia in diabetic women are the same as for non-diabetic women. Since pre-eclampsia is more common in diabetic pregnancy, however, the need for induction for this reason is greater. Proteinuria is the key indicator, but a significantly and persistently raised blood pressure alone in late pregnancy is an adequate indication by itself. Severe pre-eclampsia may, as indicated above, be best managed by caesarean section.

Essential hypertension

Essential hypertension in pregnancy presents before the onset of pregnancy and if detected prior to the 20th week may be associated with diabetic nephropathy. It may also be associated with a degree of intra-uterine growth retardation, although this can to some extent be masked by the macrosomia-inducing effect of the mother's condition. The timing of induction will depend on the progress of the condition and on the fetus. As long as the blood pressure does not rise significantly above the early pregnancy readings, there is no proteinuria and the fetal parameters of growth and wellbeing are satisfactory, induction is not indicated. A rise in blood pressure, especially if proteinuria develops or there is a definite falling off in the fetal growth pattern calls for induction or, in some cases, for elective caesarean section. Similarly, if the indicators of fetal wellbeing (biophysical profile) indicate a change in fetal condition induction is called for.

Diabetic vasculopathy

Diabetic retinopathy and nephropathy are not by themselves indications for early delivery, but their existence does impose an additional health hazard to the pregnant patient. In the case of nephropathy, pre-eclampsia is likely to be superimposed at some stage and delivery thereafter should be brought about by induction or, if severe, by planned caesarean section.

Obstetric management of labour

Induction of labour can usually be achieved by the use of a single prostaglandin pessary (PGE II, 3 mg) inserted into the posterior fornix. When contractions are established and the cervix starts to dilate simple forewater rupture ensures steady progress. Augmentation of labour, if the partograph indicates that progress is delayed, can be achieved with the cautious use of intravenous oxytocin, taking great care to avoid hyperstimulation. The fact that maternal diabetes can be well controlled by means of intravenous glucose and insulin for up to 24 hours means that there is no need to accelerate labour unduly and unnecessary augmentation should be avoided if progress is steady, even if slow. Continuous fetal heart monitoring using an external ultrasound sensor or a fetal scalp electrode is an essential part of the management of diabetic labour because of the increased risk of fetal distress (see below). Epidural analgesia has much to commend it, but there is no objection to any of the alternative forms of analgesia commonly used in labour.

Spontaneous labour

When labour starts spontaneously it is managed in the same way as induced labour, except that the need for augmentation is less likely.

Operative delivery

The decision to terminate the labour of a diabetic woman needs careful consideration by an experienced obstetrician. Delay in progress in the first or second stages, or fetal distress or difficulty in controlling maternal diabetes indicate the need to expedite delivery. Caesarean section will usually be the method of choice, but when the patient is fully dilated the question of forceps delivery arises. There is no objection to easy forceps delivery but difficult forceps delivery, bearing in mind that the baby may be big if not actually macrosomic, should be avoided because of the risk of birth trauma. This is one situation where careful assessment of a patient in the operating theatre prepared for caesarean section may be helpful. A tentative attempt at forceps delivery can be made and if an easy vaginal delivery is clearly possible caesarean section can be avoided. The advantage of an epidural analgesia in this situation is obvious. A competent neonatal paediatrician should always be present when a diabetic patient is delivered, so that paediatric care can start immediately after birth.

Fetal distress

In a series reported by Brudenell (1978) the overall incidence of fetal distress in diabetic labour was 25%. It was the commonest indication for caesarean section in labour. It was more common in primigravidas than in multigravidas. The incidence was reduced when the present regime of intravenous insulin and glucose was introduced, suggesting that the more efficient control of blood glucose levels obtained by this method rather than by intermittent subcutaneous injections of insulin was beneficial. Olofsson et al (1986) did not find a correlation between blood glucose levels and fetal distress in labour, although they confirmed a high incidence of caesarean section and low Apgar scores at birth, suggesting that fetal distress is more common in diabetic women. The association between hyperglycaemia and a raised plasma lactate and lowered plasma pH was first noticed in the anoxic sheep fetus by Shelly et al (1975), who showed that in the presence of hyperglycaemia the plasma lactate and pH changes were accentuated by hyperglycaemia. Mild hypoxia in labour in diabetic patients may, therefore, be a cause of fetal distress due to fetal anoxia in the presence of maternal and hence fetal hyperglycaemia. It is possible that fetal hyperinsulinaemia itself may be associated with an increased demand for oxygen, leading, when the demand cannot be fully met as for example in labour, to fetal hypoxia (MacFarlane & Tsakalakos 1983). Preliminary studies at King's College Hospital employing ultra-sound-directed fetal blood sampling in late pregnancy suggest that in some cases of diabetic pregnancy the fetus may be mildly hypoxic before the onset of labour and would therefore be more prone to develop fetal distress when labour starts. Further work is needed to explore this hypothesis but, for the present, the risk of fetal distress in diabetic labour may be assumed to be greater than in non-diabetic labour. Careful fetal monitoring throughout labour is clearly mandatory (see also Ch. 11).

Medical management of labour

The glucose-controlled insulin infusion is the basis of good diabetic control in labour. Blood glucose measurements should be made every hour and insulin dosage adjusted accordingly. Insulin requirements often fall in the first stage of labour. Jovanovic & Pedersen (1983) found that there was a nil requirement for insulin during the active first stage but that insulin requirement returned in the second stage. Oxytocin infusion did not affect insulin requirement and neither did epidural analgesia. Care is needed immediately after delivery when insulin requirement falls sharply, to avoid hypoglycaemia. The management of maternal diabetes in labour at King's College Hospital can be summarized as follows:

1. One litre of 5% glucose is given intravenously every 8 hours.
2. One unit of soluble insulin in 1 ml saline is administered intravenously by infusion pump. The amount of insulin given varies (normal range 0.5–2 units/h) according to the results of the hourly blood glucose estimation. The aim is to keep the blood glucose level in the range 4–6 mmol/l.
3. The regime is continued throughout labour and delivery until the mother starts to take normal meals again. As insulin requirements fall immediately after delivery, the pre-pregnancy insulin dose is given when the infusion is stopped.

The insulin infusion rate is determined as follows:

If blood glucose <4 mmol/l	0.5 U/h
If blood glucose 4–15 mmol/l	2 U/h
If blood glucose >15 mmol/l	4 U/h

(Watkins P J 1982).

After completion of the operation the regimen is continued until normal meals are taken.

The above procedure of intravenous insulin and glucose infusion is equally applicable for an emergency caesarean section as long as the guidelines for blood sugar levels are followed.

Mode of delivery

The mode of delivery at King's College Hospital in the years 1970–85 is shown in Tables 9.1 and 9.2. The actual overall caesarean section rate was much higher than in non-diabetic pregnancy. This was true for both primigravidae and multigravidae, although the rate for primigravidae was less than the overall rate. Failure of induction, fetal distress and lack of progress in labour were the main contributors to the increase in caesarean sections over the planned number. Given the problems

Table 9.1 Diabetic pregnancy. Mode of delivery at King's College Hospital

	1971–80		1981–85	
Planned C/S	123	35%	47	24%
Induction	177	50%	90	47%
Spontaneous onset	52	15%	56	29%

Table 9.2 Diabetic pregnancy—mode of delivery

	1971–80		1981–85	
Planned C/S	123	34%	47	24%
Induction—C/S	45	13%	30	16%
Spontaneous onset—C/S	11	3%	23	12%
Overall C/S rate	179	50%	110	52%
Induction—vaginal delivery	132	38%	60	31%
Spontaneous onset—vaginal delivery	41	12%	33	17%

of diabetic pregnancy and labour, delivery by caesarean section would seem to be a small price to pay by those women whose diabetic or obstetric complications make labour more hazardous.

REFERENCES

Acker D B, Sachs B P, Fredman E A 1985 Risk factors for shoulder dystocia. Obstetrics and Gynecology 66(6): 762–768

Brudenell M 1978 Delivering the baby of a diabetic mother. Proceedings of the Royal Society of Medicine 71: 207–211

Diamond M P, Entman S S, Salyer S L, Vaughan W K, Bochin 1986 Increased risk of endometritis and wound infection after caesarian section in insulin dependent diabetic women. American Journal of Obstetrics and Gynecology 155: 297–300

Drury M I 1984 Diabetes in pregnancy. Mathews Duncan revisited. Irish Journal of Medical Science 153: 144–151

Drury M I 1986 Management of pregnant diabetic care—are the pundits right? Diabetologia 29(1): 10–12

Jovanovic L, Peterson L M 1983 Insulin and glucose requirements during the first stage of labour in insulin dependent diabetic women. American Journal of Medicine 75(4): 607–612

Leslie D, Coats P M 1977 Salbutamol induced diabetic ketoacidosis. British Medical Journal 2: 768

MacFarlane C M, Tsakalakos N 1983 Relative fetal hypoxia as a contributary factor to fetal macrosomia in diabetic pregnancy. Medical Hypothesis 11: 365–374

Mølsted Pedersen L, Kuhl C 1986 Obstetric management in diabetic pregnancy: the Copenhagen experience. Diabetologia 29(1): 13–16

Murphy J, Peters J, Mossis P, Hayes T M, Pearson J F 1984 Conservative management of pregnancy in diabetic women. British Medical Journal 288: 1203–1205

Olufsson D, Ingemarsson I, Solum T 1986 Fetal distress during labour in diabetic pregnancy. British Journal of Obstetrics and Gynaecology 93(16): 1067–1071

Pearce M 1985 Management of preterm labour. In: Studd J (ed) The management of labour. Blackwell, London, pp 53–54

Shelley H J, Bassett J M, Milner R D G 1975 Control of carbohydrate metabolism in the fetus and newborn. British Medical Bulletin 31: 37–43

Stallone L A, Ziel H K 1974 Management of gestational diabetes. American Journal of Obstetrics and Gynecology 119: 1191–1194

Thomas D J B, Gill B, Brown P et al 1977 Salbutamol induced diabetic ketoacidosis. British Medical Journal 272: 438

Watkins P J 1982 Control of maternal diabetes in pregnancy and labour. ABC of diabetes. British Medical Journal 285: 717–719

10

Lung function in the infants of diabetic mothers

In the days before strict control of maternal diabetes in pregnancy was practised, obstetricians were haunted by the fear of late, unexplained intrauterine death of the fetus. Early delivery, commonly at or before 36 weeks, to avoid this occurrence produced living babies who showed a great tendency to develop the respiratory distress syndrome (RDS) secondary to hyaline membrane disease. Neonatal death from this condition was common. Paediatric neonatal care at that time was not so well developed as it is today, and this contributed to the high mortality rate of the condition amongst preterm diabetic infants. The prevalence of respiratory distress in infants of diabetic mothers has fallen sharply, as has the perinatal mortality due to this condition. Later delivery, better control of maternal diabetes and improved paediatric care have all contributed to this striking improvement. Nevertheless, respiratory distress remains a problem in those babies born preterm to diabetic mothers, especially when the maternal diabetes has been badly controlled.

The implication behind these clinical facts is that maternal diabetes in some way affects the normal maturation of the fetal lung. The ability of the newborn to inflate their lungs with the first few breaths of life depends on the presence within the lungs of pulmonary surfactant which functions by lowering surface tension within the alveoli. The major component of surfactant is phospholipid, which in turn is derived by biosynthesis from glycerol. Glucose is probably the major source of the glycerol from which the complex surfactant phospholipids are made. In the non-diabetic rat, the lung responds to raised levels of glucose, but physiological levels of insulin, by increasing glycerol production. When the insulin level is also raised no such increase occurs. In diabetic rats ketoacidosis leads to a fall in glycerol production which can be corrected by normal but not by high levels of insulin. In vitro, insulin, particularly in high concentrations, delays the maturation of cultured rat fetal lung cells, by decreasing lecithin synthesis (Gross & Smith 1977). Cortisol stimulates lecithin production by cultured fetal lung cells in vitro: this action is antagonized by insulin (Smith et al 1975). Although the precise mechanism is not understood, it is clear that fetal hyperinsulinaemia could limit or decrease the production of the essential constituents of surfactant, especially phosphatidyl glycerol and inositol (Stubbs & Stubbs 1978). This hypothesis provides an attractive explanation for the increased occurrence of respiratory distress/hyaline membrane disease in the infants of diabetic mothers who often exhibit hyperinsulinaemia. Prematurity will exaggerate the effect. Corticosteroids act as insulin antagonists, which may explain their success in preventing the development of respiratory distress in some premature infants if given to the mother prior to delivery. Fetal anoxia also suppresses surfactant production and may be an important additional factor in some cases of impaired placental function in pregnancy or complicated labour.

Measuring fetal lung maturity

Surfactant levels in the amniotic fluid reflect the levels in the fetal lung and are predictive of fetal lung maturity and the risk of respiratory distress (Whittle et al 1982). Various tests have been applied to liquor amnii obtained by amniocentesis in late pregnancy, but the one most widely used is the measurement of the lecithin : sphyngomyelin area ratio (LS). This investigation, introduced by Gluck et al (1971), has stood the test of time; an LS ratio of 2 or more is predictive of lung maturity in 99% of normal pregnant women.

At King's College Hospital the LS ratio was measured in 263 diabetic pregnancies; eight babies developed respiratory distress/hyaline membrane disease and all had an LS ratio of less than 2. There was no case of respiratory distress where the LS ratio was greater than 2. One 31-week premature baby with an LS ratio of less than 2 died. In diabetic women, however, the LS ratio may give rise to false positives, as also occurs in severe rhesus isoimmunization and birth asphyxia (Tchobroutsky et al

1978). Furthermore, an LS ratio of less than 2 does *not* mean that the baby will invariably get respiratory distress. The predictive value for RDS of an immature LS ratio (less than 2) was found to be only 50% in one series (O'Brien & Cefalo 1980).

An improvement on the predictive value of the examination of the liquor amnii came with the measurement of other phospholipids of surfactant. Phosphatidyl glycerol has proved to be the most accurate predictor of lung maturity. When it is present in the liquor respiratory distress does not occur even when the LS ratio is less than 2 (Gluck et al 1971). Using two-dimensional chromatography and measuring both LS ratio and phosphatidyl glycerol, it has been shown (Gluck et al 1971) that detectable phosphatidyl glycerol had a predictive value of lung maturity of 99% compared with 94% for a mature LS ratio. When the LS ratio was less than 2, the incidence of respiratory distress was 61%. When the LS ratio was less than 2 and phosphatidyl glycerol was absent, the incidence of RDS was 81%. In some diabetics it seems that the appearance of phosphatidyl glycerol may be delayed (Hallman & Teramo 1981).

In practice, it is best to do both tests; even if phosphatidyl glycerol is absent, a high LS ratio (greater than 3) indicates a low risk of respiratory distress. In a series of 35 diabetic pregnancies, all of whom had an LS ratio of greater than 2, four nevertheless developed respiratory distress. When phosphatidyl glycerol and lecithin concentrations were taken into account and the liquor was mature, i.e. lecithin 50 mg/l or above and phosphatidyl glycerol 2 mg/l or above, no babies out of 20 got respiratory distress, whilst 4 of 10 who gave an immature prediction did so (James et al 1984).

The measurement of actual concentrations is more laborious than the measurement of LS ratio and the simple detection of phosphatidyl glycerol, but if time allows this approach may provide a more accurate predictor of respiratory distress (Kulovich & Gluck 1979). It must be said that two variables probably affect most of these studies of liquor surfactant and respiratory distress: the technical difficulties in the actual biophysical measurements made and the difficulty in differentiating mild cases of respiratory distress from the much less serious condition of transient tachypnoea of the newborn (Brudenell, Gamsu & Roberts 1980). The variation found by different observers in both the reliability of the measurements made on the fluid and on the prevalence of respiratory distress certainly suggests that in the clinical situation the decision should be based on local experience of both. Cetrulo et al (1985), in an endeavour to avoid the difficulties associated with measuring surfactant, investigated the value of measuring the optical density of liquor at 650 nm. In a series of 428 amniotic fluids examined in this way, an optical density reading of greater than or equal to 0.15 was associated with the subsequent development of hyaline membrane disease in only two infants. The accuracy of the method was 99.53% and the false positive rate 0.47. The authors conclude that this simple and accurate test can satisfy the requirement of an on demand test of fetal pulmonary maturity.

When preterm labour is only threatened and the membranes are intact, the use of a β-agonist such as ritodrine or salbutamol is likely to be successful, at least in the short term. Once the contractions have been stopped an amniocentesis under ultrasound control should be performed and the liquor LS ratio and phosphatidyl glycerol status established. If the findings indicate that the fetal lungs are immature, a course of intramuscular dexamethasone (4 mg 8-hourly for 48 hours) or betamethasone (12 mg daily for 2 days) is likely to reduce the risk of respiratory distress if the baby is born more than 24 hours and less than 7 days after the first injection. At the end of 7 days, if actual labour has still not developed, amniocentesis and liquor examination can be repeated and a further course of steroids given if necessary. Alternatively, a weekly course of steroids may be given without repeat amniocentesis up to 34 weeks' gestation. Giving a diabetic woman corticosteroids is likely to make her hyperglycaemic unless very careful attention is paid to insulin dosage. Insulin is best given in this situation by the intravenous route, using a motorized pump. The blood glucose level should be monitored every 2 hours and insulin dosage adjusted accordingly.

When the patient is admitted with pre-term labour established, and especially if the membranes have ruptured, it is not usually worthwhile trying to stop the contractions. In this case, the neonatal intensive care unit should be warned to expect a baby that is at high risk of respiratory distress. When premature rupture of the membranes occurs before the onset of contractions it may be possible to obtain a sample of liquor either by amniocentesis or from the vaginal pool and estimate fetal lung maturity from the sample obtained. Thereafter, corticosteroids can be given if appropriate before the inevitable onset of contractions. It is usually not worthwhile trying to stop the contractions once they do start after premature rupture of the membranes, but a gap of 48 hours or more between the two events is not uncommon and allows for the possibility of accelerating fetal lung maturity.

Conclusions

The occurrence of respiratory distress in the infants of diabetic mothers has fallen sharply since the introduction of strict control of maternal diabetes in pregnancy, and in most cases it is no longer necessary to carry out tests of lung function prior to delivery. In strictly controlled diabetic pregnancies fetal lung maturation at 37 weeks and thereafter is no different from non-diabetic pregnancy (Tyden et al 1984). When delivery occurs between 32 weeks and 37 weeks respiratory complications are more likely to occur, but if maternal diabetic control has been good severe respiratory distress is uncommon. When control has been poor, delivery before 37 weeks, but especially before 32 weeks, is very likely to be complicated by respiratory distress. In such cases estimations of surfactant levels in the amniotic fluid prior to delivery provide an accurate prognostic guide and, in selective cases, indicate the need for postponing delivery until corticosteroids can be given to the mother to accelerate fetal lung maturation.

REFERENCES

Brudenell J M, Gamsu H R, Roberts A 1980 Lecithin-sphyingomyelin area ratio, respiratory distress and transient tachypnoea of the newborn. British Journal of Obstetrics and Gynaecology 87: 638

Cetrulo C L, Sbarra A J, Selarag R J et al 1985 Positive correlation between mature amniotic fluid optical density readings and the absence of neonatal hyaline membrane disease. Journal of Reproductive Medicine 30 (12): 929–932

Gluck L, Kulovich M V, Bover R C et al 1971 Diagnosis of respiratory distress syndrome by amniocentesis. American Journal of Obstetrics and Gynecology 109: 440–445

Gross I, Smith G J W 1977 Insulin delays the maturation of fetal rat lung in vitro. Paediatrics Research 11: 515–517

Hallman M, Teramo K 1981 Measurement of the lecithin/sphingomyelin ratio and phosphatidyl glycerol in amniotic fluid, an accurate method for the assessment of fetal lung maturation. British Journal of Obstetrics and Gynaecology 88: 806–813

James D K, Harkes A, Williams M et al 1984 Amniotic phosphatidyl glycerol and prediction of fetal lung maturity in diabetic pregnancies. Journal of Obstetrics and Gynecology 4: 166–169

Kulovich M V, Gluck L 1979 The lung profile. II Complicated pregnancy. American Journal of Obstetrics and Gynecology 135: 64–70

O'Brien W F, Cefalo R C 1980 Clinical applicability of amniotic fluid tests for fetal pulmonary maturity. American Journal of Obstetrics and Gynecology 136: 135–144

Smith B, Girond C, Robert M, Avery M E 1975 Insulin antagonism of cortisol action on lecithin synthesis by cultured fetal lung cells. Journal of Pediatrics 87: 953

Stubbs W A, Stubbs S M 1978 Hyperinsulinaemia diabetes mellitus and respiratory distress of the newborn, a common link? Lancet i: 308–309

Tchbroutsky C, Amiel-Tison C, Cedard L et al 1978 The lecithin-sphyingomyelin ratio in 132 insulin-dependent diabetic pregnancies. American Journal of Obstetrics and Gynecology 130: 754–760

Tyden O, Berne C, Eriksson U J et al 1984 Fetal maturation in strictly controlled diabetic pregnancy. Diabetes Research Sept Col 1 (3): 131–134

Whittle M J, Wilson A I, Whitfield C R et al 1982 An amniotic fluid phospholipid profile determined by two-dimensional layer chromatography as an index of fetal lung maturation. British Journal of Obstetrics and Gynaecology 89: 727–732

11
Perinatal and maternal mortality

The most significant aspect of diabetic pregnancy in recent years has been the fall in perinatal mortality. Although in specialized units the rate approaches that found in non-diabetic pregnancy, overall the risk to the fetus of a diabetic mother is still increased several fold. Perinatal morbidity is also raised, so that the short-term outlook for an infant of a diabetic mother is less favourable than in non-diabetic pregnancy and there may be some long-term disadvantages too, although these are not generally serious.

An analysis of the cause of perinatal mortality in diabetic pregnancy is useful, since it provides a basis for rational clinical management. It is convenient to consider perinatal mortality under five separate headings, shown in Table 11.1. This table also illustrates the changing pattern of mortality during the 35-year period at King's. The figures include all babies delivered, whether booked, i.e. seen in the antenatal clinic before 20 weeks, or unbooked, i.e. late (after 20 weeks) referrals from other hospitals.

Table 11.1 Diabetic pregnancies—King's College Hospital

		Causes of perinatal mortality—1951–85				
	No.	Perinatal deaths	Obstet.[a]	Diab.[b]	Cong[c] abn.	RDS[d]	Unexplained
1951–60	319	72 (22.5%)	26	5	6	17	18
1961–70	390	39 (10.0%)	9	2	5	8	15
1971–80	352	13 (3.7%)	3	1	6	1	2
1981–85	193	2 (1.0%)	0	0	2	0	0

[a] Obstetric.
[b] Diabetic.
[c] Congenital abnormality.
[d] Respiratory distress syndrome.

'Unexplained' perinatal mortality

This category refers, very largely, to intrauterine death occurring without warning during the last 4–6 weeks of pregnancy. In the early part of the 1951–70 period some babies died within the first 24 hours of life of profound hypoglycaemia, then insufficiently recognized and badly treated. Once this problem was recognized and early effective treatment instituted, neonatal death from this cause ceased to be a problem. Indeed the whole category of unexplained perinatal deaths, as shown in the table, has diminished considerably in the past 15 years.

The importance of unexplained late intrauterine fetal death is not so much the magnitude of the fetal risk, which nowadays is very small, but the influence which it has had on the clinical management of diabetic pregnancy. To obviate this once serious risk, premature delivery was and is still widely practised. Babies who were delivered by caesarean section at 35–36 weeks often died in the neonatal period of respiratory distress as a result. Once the importance of proper control of maternal diabetes was recognized the risk of late intrauterine death receded rapidly, but even so many diabetic pregnancies are still terminated before term as a precaution.

It may, of course, be argued that late intrauterine death has disappeared simply because diabetic pregnancies have not been allowed to go to full term and that if they all were the problem would arise again. It is impossible to refute this argument completely, although in recent times a number of reports have shown that, in well-controlled diabetics, allowing pregnancy to proceed to full term and beyond is not harmful to the normally grown fetus. Caution is needed before adopting this policy across the board, however, for developing fetal macrosomia means that a particular fetus is being affected by the maternal diabetes even though this is well controlled. In such cases the risk of unexplained intrauterine death is higher and preterm delivery, usually at 37–38 weeks, is indicated.

The cause of late intrauterine death has until recently been unexplained. A consideration of the factors involved in fetal oxygenation in diabetic pregnancy leads to the conclusion that the cause is fetal anoxia. Blood flow *to* the intervillus space is normal in uncomplicated diabetic pregnancy (Brudenell et al 1961). However, radioactive clearance studies (Rekonen et al 1976, Anderson et al 1985) have indicated that blood flow *through* the intervillus space may be reduced by as much as 35–45%. This reduction in flow is likely to result from morphological changes in the diabetic placenta, in particular villous oedema, increased branching of the villi and an increase in the fetal intravillous blood volume (see Ch. 14). These and other changes will also hinder oxygen transfer to the fetus from the maternal blood. HbA_{1c} has an increased affinity for oxygen, so releases it less actively than normal HbA. In badly-controlled diabetic pregnancy, raised levels of HbA_{1c} may decrease oxygen release by as much as 10% (Madsden & Ditzel 1982, 1984). The consumption of oxygen by the diabetic fetus and placenta is increased in the presence of hyperinsulinaemia (Carson et al 1980, Milley et al 1984). Hypoxia in the presence of hyperglycaemia leads to an increased metabolism of glucose through the hexose monophosphate shunt pathway, resulting in an exaggerated synthesis of and deposition of triglycerides in the fetal adipose tissue, so increasing fetal macrosomia (MacFarlane & Tsakalakos 1983).

The combination of impaired delivery of oxygen to the placenta, an impaired transfer of oxygen to the fetus and increased fetal and placental consumption point to a degree of fetal hypoxia in diabetic pregnancy. This is not severe in the well-controlled, uncomplicated case but may become so in the presence of maternal vascular disease, hypertension or pre-eclampsia and when the mother is badly controlled. Maternal ketoacidosis is especially harmful to normal oxygenation because of the effect it has on the oxygen dissociation curve. Relative hypoxia in the fetus leads to an increased incidence of fetal distress in labour (Brudenell 1978) and neonatal asphyxia, and is responsible for the polycythaemia and subsequent jaundice seen in the infant of the diabetic mother. Until recently, direct evidence of relative hypoxia in the diabetic fetus has been lacking. Cordocentesis under direct ultrasound control allows samples of fetal blood to be obtained at various stages of pregnancy. A preliminary study at King's College Hospital (Brudenell 1987) on 16 diabetic pregnancies has confirmed that even in the well-controlled diabetic pregnancy a degree of hypoxia exists in the fetus. Thus hypoxia is the probable cause of late intrauterine fetal death in diabetic pregnancy and is most likely to occur when the pregnancy is complicated or badly controlled and the fetus macrosomic.

Obstetric causes of perinatal mortality

Table 11.2 shows the perinatal deaths which occurred as a result of obstetric complications. The fall in this previously important cause of perinatal mortality during the past 15 years in fact reflects the improvement in obstetric care generally, but also represents the advantages that accrue from better control of the maternal diabetes. This is particularly true of the incidence of pre-eclampsia and hydramnios; although these complications are still more common in diabetic pregnancy in the UK generally (Beard & Lowy 1982), they are much less common than previously and should not represent an increased risk for the fetus when maternal control is good. Birth trauma as a cause of perinatal mortality results directly from fetal macrosomia causing difficulties in delivery. The possibility that a traumatic delivery may cause perinatal death or morbidity must always be borne in mind when delivering a diabetic woman, particularly if there is any suggestion of fetal macrosomia or indeed any other cause of disproportion. Difficult vaginal deliveries have no place in the management of diabetic pregnancy. The remaining obstetric complications shown in the table are no more likely to occur in diabetic than in non-diabetic pregnancy; they serve as a reminder that in diabetic pregnancy, problems unrelated to the maternal diabetes may be equally dangerous to the fetus.

Table 11.2 Obstetric causes of perinatal death

	1951–70	*1971–85*
Birth trauma	9	0
Pre-eclampsia	9	0
APH	4	3
Acute hydramnios	4	0
IUGR	3	0
Intrapartum asphyxia	3	0
Rhesus incompatibility	2	0
Other	8	0

'Diabetic' causes of perinatal mortality

It has long been recognized that true diabetic coma with ketoacidosis in insulin-dependent diabetics causes intrauterine death of the fetus. The severity of the maternal biochemical upset which will kill the fetus varies considerably, but in any diabetic pregnant woman the development of ketoacidosis puts the fetus immediately at risk; presumably this is because it is unable to maintain its own biochemical balance in the face of ketone bodies which pass freely across the placenta. The prevalence of this cause of stillbirth in diabetic pregnancy has diminished sharply in recent years and has only been seen twice at King's College Hospital in over 600 diabetic pregnancies since 1970. Both cases were unbooked and were transferred into the unit in established ketoacidosis, with the fetus already dead. One of the cases occurred in an intelligent diabetic woman who preferred to manage her own diabetes and did not sufficiently appreciate the change in requirements for insulin in pregnancy. This might not have mattered too much, but at 30 weeks she developed an abscess in her neck: she failed to seek medical advice, became ill with the infection and quickly lapsed into diabetic ketoacidosis, in which state she was admitted to hospital. Rapid control of the diabetes was achieved with intravenous insulin and glucose but the fetus was already dead and was delivered in a macerated state some days later.

All pregnant diabetic women need to be aware of the increased difficulty in maintaining strict control in pregnancy and should be able to contact their medical advisers immediately they suspect the control is slipping. That those same advisers need to be equally vigilant is illustrated by a case that occurred in the 1951–70 series. The patient, an insulin-dependent diabetic at 26 weeks' gestation, was an inpatient being treated for persistent pregnancy vomiting. The vomiting suddenly increased during one weekend and the patient went into coma because the locum house physician did not recognize the danger promptly. On Monday morning the patient was severely ketoacidotic and the fetus had died in utero. This sort of accident should not occur nowadays with easily applied methods of determining blood glucose levels, both on a do-it-yourself basis in the patient's own home, with either a glucose meter or B-M stix, and in the antenatal or labour ward of the hospital. First class and accurate biochemical laboratory back up is essential in the latter setting for dealing with established cases of coma, but it is the initial measurement of the blood glucose level and testing the urine for ketones by the patient or physician at the slightest sign of loss of control that is important if the fetus is to escape from the threat posed by maternal ketoacidosis.

Maternal hypoglycaemia has traditionally been regarded as not being harmful to the fetus. Since these hypoglycaemic attacks are usually only transient and result from overdosage of insulin in an attempt to achieve an especially good control, no demonstrable harm is done to the fetus. However, if the fetus has been rendered hyperinsulinaemic by chronic maternal hyperglycaemia, an episode of hypoglycaemia could, theoretically, contribute to profound and possibly fatal fetal hypoglycaemia.

It is clear that if perinatal mortality and morbidity are to be avoided the best possible control of the maternal diabetes is essential, so that both extremes of the glycaemic range are avoided.

Respiratory distress and perinatal mortality

Respiratory distress results from the formation of hyaline membrane in the lungs, which in turn is caused by deficient production of surfactant (see Ch. 10). The infants of diabetic mothers have traditionally been more prone to this condition, particularly when maternal diabetes has been badly controlled and the baby delivered prematurely. The dramatic fall in perinatal mortality from this cause over the past 15 years has been due to a number of factors. Good maternal diabetic control certainly helps to keep fetal lung surfactant production up to nondiabetic fetal levels, and it is possible to measure such levels of production by estimating levels of various surfactants, especially lecithin, sphyngomyelin and phosphatidyl glycerol, in the liquor amnii in late pregnancy. The ability to do this whenever preterm delivery is contemplated in diabetic pregnancy has been especially valuable in indicating the need to delay delivery when surfactant levels are less than optimum. Latterly confidence at King's College Hospital has grown to the extent that amniocentesis is no longer performed after 34 weeks unless the maternal diabetic control has been bad. (Before 32 weeks attempts are usually made to accelerate pulmonary maturation using corticosteroids.) This confidence stems not only from the knowledge that good control renders respiratory distress unlikely, but also from the very considerable advances made by neonatal paediatricians in its treatment. Delivery by caesarean section has been held to be an aetiological factor in respiratory distress but the evidence is unconvincing, so a high caesarean section rate in diabetic pregnancy will not cause a high incidence of this condition. Fetal anoxia in labour is a more important contributing factor to respiratory distress and is particularly to be avoided in diabetic women in labour from this, as well as other, important points of view.

Congenital abnormality in perinatal mortality

Congenital abnormality remains an important cause of perinatal mortality: as will be seen in Table 11.1, the incidence of this cause of perinatal loss did not change in the 30-year period between 1951 and 1980 but with the decrease in deaths from other causes it has become relatively much more important. The increased incidence of congenital abnormality in diabetic pregnancy implies that some aspect of the diabetic woman's 'milieu interieur' is harmful to the developing embryo. The subject is considered in more detail in Chapter 12.

Maternal mortality in diabetic pregnancy

The general fall in maternal mortality for all pregnancies is reflected in the fall in maternal mortality in diabetic pregnancy, so that it is now extremely rare for a diabetic woman to die as a result of pregnancy. The very low present day maternal mortality figures in diabetic pregnancy are in striking contrast to the 45% maternal mortality in 66 diabetic pregnancies reported on by Williams in 1909. It is generally held that diabetic women are at greater risk than non-diabetic women, but there are no accurate figures to support this contention. There were no maternal deaths in a series of 600 diabetic pregnancies reported by Drury (1977) or in the 1403 diabetic pregnancies in the British Diabetic Pregnancy Survey (Beard & Lowy 1982). The only maternal death associated with diabetic pregnancy at King's College Hospital in the 15 years from 1971–1986 occurred in a patient with advanced diabetic nephropathy who died from renal failure 11 months after successful delivery. Seven maternal deaths in diabetic pregnancy were reported in the reports on Confidential Enquiries into Maternal Deaths in England and Wales (1976–81).

Maternal deaths in diabetic pregnancy in England and Wales 1976–81

1. Badly-controlled 27-year-old insulin-dependent diabetic. Delivered by caesarean section at 32 weeks because of acute hydramnios. Died in operating theatre. Autopsy revealed severe coronary atheroma causing myocardial infarction.
2. Badly-controlled 19-year-old insulin-dependent diabetic. Admitted to hospital at 29 weeks in diabetic ketoacidotic coma. Autopsy revealed pneumonia and empyema.
3. Glycosuria detected at 34 weeks in a 26-year-old para 4. Admitted in premature labour before investigations could be started and went into ketoacidotic coma after delivery. Died 1 day post partum of disseminated intravascular coagulation and septicaemia complicating diabetes.
4. Insulin-dependent diabetic admitted to hospital at 11 weeks because of persistent nausea and vomiting. Three weeks later, whilst still in hospital, had a cardiac arrest attributed to severe hypoglycaemia.
5. Badly-controlled insulin-dependent diabetic developed diabetic ketoacidosis at 25 weeks. Pregnancy terminated by hysterotomy. Patient died on 13th postoperative day from bronchopneumonia.
6. Primigravida aged 38 with a long-standing insulin-dependent diabetes complicated by severe hypertension. Elective caesarean section at 38 weeks. Died following cardiac arrest, cause unknown, during induction of anaesthesia.
7. A badly-controlled obese diabetic had a pulmonary embolism at 28 weeks. Treated with heparin. Preterm labour 4 days later led to spontaneous vaginal delivery. Massive pulmonary embolus caused death 40 days after delivery, the patient having cooperated poorly in her anticoagulant and diabetic treatment.

The only general conclusion that can be drawn from this series is that poor diabetic control is the major factor contributing to the maternal death in most cases. Loss of diabetic control leading to ketoacidosis threatens the mother as well as the fetus, although the risk to the latter is much greater. The practical point that again emerges is that patients must be quick to report at once any loss of diabetic control, however slight, to the combined diabetic antenatal clinic. Good communications between patient and diabetic physician are the key to the prevention of diabetic ketoacidosis. Similarly, when pregnant patients are admitted to hospital with difficulties in controlling their diabetes, immediate specialist care is needed, usually involving an intravenous insulin regime. Long-standing diabetics with known vascular disease should understand the additional risks they run if they embark on a pregnancy and will often best be advised not to do so.

REFERENCES

Anderson K V, Hermann N, Munch O, Larsen J F 1985 Intervillous blood flow in the human placenta. Ugeskrift for Laegar 147: 1018–1024

Beard R W, Lowy C 1982 British survey of diabetic pregnancies. British Journal of Obstetrics and Gynaecology 89: 783–786

Brudenell J M 1978 Delivering the infant of a diabetic mother. Proceedings of the Royal Society of Medicine 71: 211–221

Brudenell J M 1987 Observations on fetal cord blood PO_2 in diabetic pregnancy. William Meredith Fletcher Shaw Memorial Lecture. Royal College of Obstetricians and Gynaecologists.

Brudenell J M, Miles J M, Coleman A 1961 The clearance of radioactive sodium from the myometrium of the pregnant diabetic. Journal of Obstetrics and Gynaecology of the British Commonwelth 68: 238–246

Carson B S, Phillips A F, Simons M A, Ballaglea F C, Meschia G 1980 Effects of a sustained insulin infusion upon glucose uptake and oxygenation of the ovine fetus. Pediatric Research 14: 147–152

Drury M I, Green A T, Stronge J M 1977 Pregnancy complicated by clinical diabetes mellitus. Obstetrics and Gynecology 49: 519

MacFarlane C M, Tsakalakos N 1983 Relative fetal hypoxia as a contributing factor to fetal macrosomia in diabetic pregnancy. Medical Hypothesis 11: 365–374

Madsden H, Ditzel J 1982 Changes in red cell oxygen transport in diabetic pregnancy. American Journal of Obstetrics and Gynecology 143: 421–424

Madsden H, Ditzel J 1984 Blood oxygen transport in the first trimester of diabetic pregnancy. Acta Obstetrica and Gynecologica Scandinavia 63: 312–320

Milley J R, Rosenberg A A, Phillips A F, Molteni R A, Jones M D, Simmons M A 1984 The effect of insulin on fetal oxygen exchange. American Journal of Obstetrics and Gynecology 149: 673–678

Rekonen A, Luotola H, Pitkänen M, Kinkka J, Pyorala J 1976 Measurement of intervillous and myometrial blood flow by an intravenous [113]Xe method. British Journal of Obstetrics and Gynaecology 83: 723–728

Report on Confidential Enquiries into Maternal Deaths in England and Wales 1976–1985 and 1979–1981. Her Majesty's Stationery Office, London, pp. 119 and 97

Williams J W 1909 The clinical significance of glycosuria in pregnant women. American Journal of Medical Science 137: 1

12

Congenital abnormality

As noted in Chapter 6, congenital abnormality is now the most important contributor to perinatal mortality and morbidity in diabetic pregnancy. Early workers in the field questioned whether or not there was a real increase in the frequency of congenital malformations, but in the past 20 years the association has been clearly established. It is now accepted that the diabetic woman is three to four times more likely to have a congenitally malformed baby than her non-diabetic counterpart (Malins 1979, Mølsted-Pederson 1980, Fuhrmann et al 1983). Lowy et al (1986), reporting on the UK diabetic pregnancy survey, showed that the malformation rate in IDD was 7.1% and for NIDD, 1.9%. This is in accord with our experience at King's (Table 12.1), which also illustrates the range of abnormalities. Table 12.2 illustrates the contribution which fatal congenital malformations have made to perinatal mortality during the 35 years, 1951–85. To the clinician, the interest lies in two aspects; *a*) what

Table 12.1 Diabetic pregnancy in King's College Hospital 1971–85: major congenital abnormalities

CNS	11
Skeletal	10
Cardiac	9
Alimentary	3
Caudal regression	2
Multiple	2
Hypoplastic lungs	1
Potters syndrome	1
Total	39
Prevalence	39/545 (7.2%)

Table 12.2   Diabetic pregnancies in King's College Hospital 1951–85

	No	Perinatal deaths	Fatal congenital malformations		TOP* for congenital malformations
1951–60	318	72	6	8%	—
1961–60	389	39	5	13%	—
1971–80	352	13	6	46%	5
1981–85	193	2	2	100%	3

* Termination of pregnancy

causes the abnormalities and *b*) can good diabetic control decrease the incidence of abnormality?

The cause of congenital abnormality in diabetic pregnancy

The most important time for diabetic control during organogenesis is the first 7 weeks of intrauterine life because it is during this period that abnormal carbohydrate metabolism might cause abnormality (Mills et al 1979). In the female rat with streptozotocin-induced diabetes pregnancy results in a high incidence of congenital abnormality, especially visceral eversion and incomplete ossification of the sacrum (Deuchar 1979). The latter anomaly is particularly significant because of its similarity to sacral agenesis/caudal regression seen in humans. Eriksson & Styrund (1985), reporting similar malformations in diabetic rats, also noted an association between sacral malformations and micrognathia similar to the femoral hypoplasia/unusual facies syndrome described by Riedel et al (1985) in the infant of a diabetic mother. Freinkel et al (1986) examined various types of fuel mediated teratogenesis during organogenesis in different species and concluded that teratogenic vulnerability may be, at least in part, genetically determined.

Although hyperglycaemia and ketoacidosis are probably the main factors, other factors indicating gene deficiency may also be important. Experimental ketoacidosis in mice causes chromosomal abnormalities with and without manifest deformities (Enricho & Ingalls 1968), so the effect of maternal diabetes may be upon the chromosomes of the oocyte or the pre- or post-implantation embryo. Hod et al (1986) reported growth retardation and dysmorphogenesis in the rat conceptus in the presence of hyperglycaemia. Sorbitol accumulated in the conceptus during the hyperglycaemia but total protein, DNA and free myoinositol decreased. Aldose reductase inhibitors prevented the rise in sorbitol but not the fall in protein, DNA and myoinositol. The rise in sorbitol consequent upon hyperglycaemia does not contribute to its adverse effects on the embryo. This finding was confirmed in a study by Eriksson et al (1986), who measured the sorbitol levels in the offspring of diabetic rats. There was no difference in the sorbitol content of the normal and abnormal offspring.

Once the embryo is implanted and starts to develop, a direct effect on the process of organogenesis is possible. Since most pregnant diabetic women do not become ketoacidotic in early pregnancy, hyperglycaemia seems the most important factor in human pregnancy. Experimental support for this suggestion comes from Sadler (1980), who showed a high rate of exencephaly in early mouse embryos grown in hyperglycaemic tissue culture, and from the preventative effect which meticulous control of maternal hyperglycaemia during organogenesis in diabetic rats has upon the incidence of congenital sacral abnormalities (Baker, Egler & Klein 1981). An increase in yolk sac failure, leading to congenital abnormality in rat conceptuses subjected to hyperglycaemia in culture, was reported by Pinter et al (1986), who emphasize the importance of a well functioning yolk sac during the period of organogenesis.

Goldman et al (1985), investigating the mechanism by which diabetes exerts its teratogenic effects, studied the effects of arachidonic acid supplementation in rats and mice. They showed that arachidonic acid exerts a significant protective effect against the teratogenic action of hyperglycaemia both in vivo (rat) and in vitro (mouse) animal models. They postulate that hyperglycaemia involves a functional deficiency of arachidonic acid at a critical stage of organogenesis. Although there is as yet no evidence to support this hypothesis in the human, it does offer a possible explanation for the increased incidence of congenital abnormality in diabetic pregnancy.

The effect of good diabetic control on the incidence of abnormality. Since the first 7 weeks of pregnancy are vital, it is clear that if the effects of maternal diabetes on organogenesis are to be mitigated the patient should be well controlled *before* conception and that good control should continue throughout the first trimester. There is good evidence that abnormality occurs less frequently in well-controlled diabetics (Pederson 1979, Fuhrmann 1983) and it has long been recognized that diabetic mothers with vascular complications, i.e. 'severe' diabetics, are more prone to have abnormal babies (Baker et al 1981). Even a mild abnormality of carbohydrate metabolism (i.e. impaired glucose tolerance in modern parlance) may be associated with an increased risk of abnormality (Tallarigo et al 1986).

Fuhrmann et al (1983), by applying very strict criteria for good diabetic control before and during pregnancy, showed a reduction of malformation to 0.8% (one case) in 128 diabetic women who had both pre- and post-conception care. In a further group of 292 women whose care started after 8 weeks, gestation there were 22 malformed infants (7.5%). The measures adopted by Fuhrmann included very frequent visits to the diabetic clinic and a high incidence of hospital in-patient care. In the pre- and post-conception care group patients were admitted every 3 months before conception for supervision of their control and as soon as body temperature elevation in the second half of the menstrual cycle indicated the possibility of pregnancy. The length of hospitalization varied for individual patients, the aim being to keep plasma glucose levels at 3.3–7.2 mmol/l.

The emergence of HbA_1 estimation as a means of judging diabetic control retrospectively has shed further light on the question of the effect of hyperglycaemia on fetal development in the first trimester. Since HbA_1 levels reflect to some extent the blood glucose concentrations during the preceding 4–6 weeks, it might be expected that those patients with a low HbA_1 level at 12 weeks' gestation would have a lower risk of having an abnormal baby than those with a high level. Taking 12% of HbA_1 measured by electrophoresis (Corning) as the dividing line between low and high there is good support for this concept (Ylinen, Raivio & Teramo 1981, Miller et al 1981, Stubbs et al 1986) which, therefore, has important practical implications. It must, however, be recognized that a normal HbA_1 level in early pregnancy may still be associated with abnormality. Mills et al (1988) examined glycaemic control in diabetic pregnancy during organogenesis and could not demonstrate a relationship between glycosylated haemoglobin or blood glucose levels and congenital malformation. They concluded that more sensitive methods are needed to identify the teratogenic mechanism.

Hypoglycaemia was not thought to be teratogenic but Buchanan et al (1986) demonstrated that pregnant diabetic rats made severely hypoglycaemic in early pregnancy had an increased incidence of dysmorphic lesions suggesting that both hypo- and hyperglycaemia should be avoided during organogenesis. Insulin is not thought to be teratogenic although the work on rumpless-ness in chickens (see p 107) is of interest. Other causes of congenital abnormality—teratogenic drugs, alcohol and rubella may operate in diabetic pregnancy. No diabetic woman should become pregnant until she is immune to rubella.

Preventing congenital abnormality in diabetic pregnancy

All diabetic women should be made aware of the need for preconception counselling so as to ensure that their diabetes is well controlled from the very start of the pregnancy. Diabetic clinics, physicians and obstetricians seeing non-diabetic women should take the opportunity to press this point (Watkins P 1982). In dealing with those women who report to the clinic when already pregnant, those who are most at risk should be recognized: they include the badly-controlled, the long-standing insulin-dependent diabetic with vascular complications and the women who have previously had an abnormal baby. A high HbA_1 level during the first 12 weeks or at the 12th week (>12%) should alert the obstetrician, since such high levels are associated with an increased risk of abnormality. The risks are relative, however, and as indicated above the majority of women with badly controlled diabetes and high HbA_1 levels in early pregnancy will have normal babies.

Detecting congenital abnormalities

Until the advent of ultrasound, diagnosis of congenital abnormality was confined to those cases with gross physical signs in mid- or late pregnancy, the diagnosis being confirmed by X-ray. Ultrasound scanning has made possible much earlier detection and the opportunity to offer the mother termination if the abnormality is severe. In the years 1981–85, of the six major congenital abnormalities in 193 babies at King's College Hospital, four were diagnosed by ultrasound, of which three were aborted. Ultrasound failed to detect one baby with an absent radius, deformed thumbs and hemivertebra and one baby with Potter's syndrome.

It has been suggested that delayed fetal growth in very early pregnancy (between 7 and 14 weeks) may indicate fetal abnormality (Pedersen & Mølsted-Pedersen 1981), but care is needed in the interpretation of early growth patterns since these may be affected by the time of ovulation and conception even when the menstrual pattern is regular and the date of the last menstrual period certain (Little et al 1981). In a more recent paper, Mølsted-Pedersen and Pedersen (1985) reported early growth delay in 7 of 9 infants of diabetic mothers with major congenital malformation. It is clearly important, therefore, that early delay in fetal growth, especially in severe or badly controlled diabetics, be taken as an indication that the full fetal anomaly scan at 18–20 weeks should be performed with the increased possibility of fetal abnormality very much in mind. When a serious congenital anomaly is detected careful counselling of the patient is needed and a neonatal paediatrician should be involved so that the nature and the effectiveness of any corrective procedures that may be possible can be discussed. This is particularly true of cardiovascular anomalies, which may be able to be corrected surgically in the early neonatal period. Such babies should be delivered in a hospital with immediate access to a specialized neonatal cardiac surgical unit (Allan et al 1986). Even severe anomalies such as sacral agenesis may be improved to a remarkable extent by corrective surgery (Fig. 12.1). In general, however, when faced with the prospect of a very abnormal baby most parents will opt for termination of pregnancy coupled with a decision either not to become pregnant again or, if a further pregnancy is contemplated, to ensure that preconception diabetic control is of a very high standard.

Transient hypertrophic sub-aortic stenosis

Gutgesell et al (1976) described three cases of this type of cardiac abnormality in three infants of diabetic mothers. The stenosis produces a form of functional left ventricular outflow obstruction which seems to resolve during the first 6 months of life. The importance of the lesion is that the infant becomes ill shortly after birth with respiratory distress and congestive heart failure resistant to digoxin and diuretics. The diagnosis is based on the

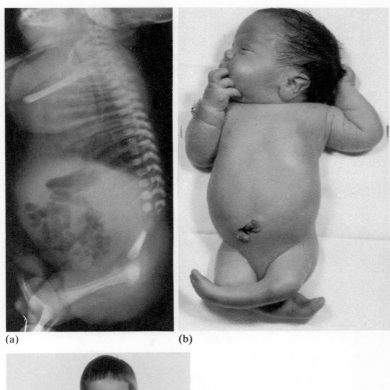

(a) (b)

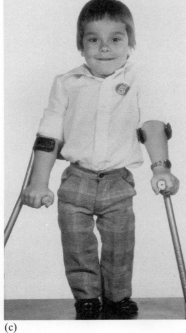

(c)

Fig. 12.1 a & b Sacral agenesis (caudal regression syndrome) in the infant of a diabetic mother. c. With corrective surgery, even sacral agenesis is compatible with a happy life

finding of a harsh systolic murmur heard to the left of the sternum, and haemodynamic and angiographic evidence of hypertrophic cardiomyopathy with outflow obstruction. The aetiology of the condition and why it should occur in the infants of diabetic mothers is not clear, but it is possible that it results from asymmetrical cardiac hypertrophy, part of the generalized organomegaly seen in these infants. Echocardiography is used to identify the condition after birth and to follow its resolution. The condition should be borne in mind if ultrasonography in pregnancy indicates cardiac enlargement or evidence of cardiac failure.

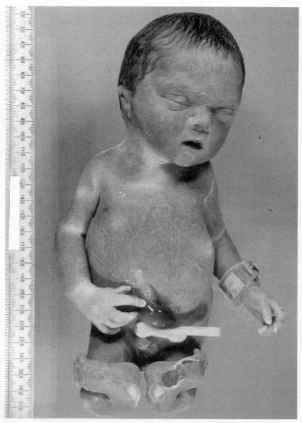

Fig. 12.2 Severe limb deformity resulting from maternal diabetes

Caudal regression syndrome (caudal dysplasia syndrome)

This congenital abnormality, described by Hohl in 1852, is rare and consists of absence of vertebrae from any level below T10 and the consequent deformities. If the sacrum is missing (sacral agenesis) the transverse diameter of the pelvis is reduced, the buttocks are flattened and there is muscular atrophy in the legs. There may be dislocation of the hips, talipes, spina bifida, renal anomalies and urinary and faecal incontinence. Lesser degrees of abnormality of the lower limbs not amounting to true caudal regression are also seen (Fig. 12.2). The caudal regression syndrome is akin to 'rumplessness' in chickens. This abnormality occurs as an hereditary condition or spontaneously. More interestingly, it can be produced experimentally in white leghorn chickens by injecting insulin into the incubating eggs. This suggests that either insulin itself or the hypoglycaemia produced by it may be teratogenic. Clinically, neither insulin nor hypoglycaemia have been thought to be important but the work of Buchanan et al (1986) suggests that, on occasion, severe hypoglycaemia may be teratogenic. The caudal regression syndrome does not occur only in IDD its incidence in diabetic pregnancy does seem to be considerably higher. The estimates of incidence in diabetic pregnancy vary widely but it is probably of the order of 1 in 1000 (Leny & Maier 1964). This level accords with the experience of King's College Hospital in recent years. Any woman giving birth to a baby showing the caudal regression syndrome who is not a known diabetic should have a glucose tolerance test.

The combined approach of prevention and early detection of congenital abnormality and selected termination in diabetic pregnancy should ensure a decrease in this cause of perinatal mortality and morbidity.

REFERENCES

Allan L D, Crawford D C, Chitra S K, Tynan M J 1986 Prenatal screening for congenital heart disease. British Medical Journal 292: 1717–1719
Baker L, Egler J M, Klein S H, Goldman A S 1981 Meticulous control of diabetes during organogenesis prevents congenital lumbo-sacral defects in rats. Diabetes 30: 955–959
Buchanan T A, Freinkel N, Schemmer J K 1986 Material insulin impairs embryo development in the rat: implications for diabetic control in early pregnancy. Diabetes: 35 Suppl. 1, 47A

Deuchar E M 1979 Experimental evidence relating fetal abnormalities to diabetes. In: Sutherland H W, Stowers J M (eds) Carbohydrate metabolism in pregnancy and the newborn. Springer Verlag, Berlin, Heidelberg, New York, pp 247–263

Enricho A, Ingalls T M 1968 Chromosomal anomalies in the embryos of diabetic mice. Archives of Environmental Health 16: 316–325

Eriksson U J, Styrund J 1985 Congenital malformations in diabetic pregnancy, the clinical relevance of experimental studies. Acta Paediatrica Scandinavia Supplement 320: 72–78

Eriksson U J, Naeser P, Brolin S E 1986 Increased accumulation of sorbitol in offspring of manifest diabetic rats. Diabetes 35 (12): 1356–1363

Freinkel N, Cockcroft D L, Lewis N J et al 1986 Fuel mediated teratogenesis during organogenesis: the effects of increased concentrations of glucose, ketones or somatomedin inhibitor during rat embryo culture. American Journal of Clinical Nutrition 44: 986–995

Fuhrmann K, Reiher H, Semmler K, Fischer F, Fischer M, Glockner E 1983 Prevention of congenital malformations in infants of insulin-dependent diabetic mothers. Diabetes Care 6: 219–223

Goldman A S, Baker L, Piddington R, Marx B, Harold R, Egler J 1985 Hyperglycaemia induced teratogenesis is mediated by a functional deficiency of arachidonic acid. Proceedings of the National Academy of Sciences of the USA 82 (23): 8227–8231

Gutgesell H P, Mullins C E, Gillett P C, Beer M, Rudolph A, MacNamara D G 1976 Transient hypertrophic sub aortic stenosis in infants of diabetic mothers. Journal of Pediatrics 89: 120–125

Hod M, Star S, Passoneau J V, Unterman T C, Freinkel N 1986 Effect of hyperglycaemia on sorbitol and myoinositol content of cultured rat conceptus. Biochemical and Biophysical Research Communications 140 (3): 974–980

Hohl A F 1852 Zur Pathologie des Beckens bl. W Engleman, Leipzig

Leny W, Maier W 1964 Congenital malformations and maternal diabetes. Lancet ii: 1124

Little D J, Stubbs S M, Brudenell M, Campbell S 1981 Early growth retardation in diabetic pregnancy. British Medical Journal 283: 488

Lowy C, Beard R W, Goldschmidt J 1986 The UK diabetic pregnancy survey. Acta Endocrinologica (Supplement) 277: 86–89

Malins J 1979 Fetal anomalies related to carbohydrate metabolism: the epidemiological approach. In: Sutherland H W, Stowers J M (eds) Carbohydrate metabolism in pregnancy and the newborn. Springer Verlag, Berlin, Heidelberg, New York, pp 229–246

Miller E, Hare J W, Cloherty J P et al 1981 Elevated maternal HbA_{1c} in early pregnancy and major congenital abnormalities in infants of diabetic mothers. New England Journal of Medicine 304: 1331–1334

Mills J L, Baker L, Goldman A S 1979 Malformations in infants of diabetic mothers occur before the 7th gestational week. Implications for treatment. Diabetes 28: 292–293

Mills J L, Knopp R H, Simpson J L et al 1988 Lack of relation of increased malformation rates in infants of diabetic mothers to glycaemic control during organogenesis. New England Medical Journal 318: 671–676

Mølsted-Pedersen L 1980 Pregnancy and diabetes, a survey. Acta Endocrinologica 94 (suppl 283): 13–19

Mølsted-Pedersen L, Pedersen J F 1985 Congenital malformations in diabetic pregnancies. Clinical viewpoints. Acta Pediatrica Scandinavia (Supplement) 320: 79–84

Pedersen J 1979 Congenital malformations in newborns of diabetic mothers. In: Sutherland H W, Stowers J M (eds) Carbohydrate metabolism in pregnancy and the newborn. Springer Verlag, Berlin, Heidelberg, New York, pp 264–276

Pedersen J F, Mølsted-Pedersen L 1981 Early fetal growth delay detected by ultrasound marks increased risk of congenital malformation in diabetic pregnancy. British Medical Journal 283: 269–271

Pinter E, Reece E A, Leranth C Z, Sanyal M K, Hobbins J G, Mahoney M J, Naftolin F 1986 Yolk sac failure in embryopathy due to hyperglycaemia. Teratology 33 (1): 73–84

Reidel F, Froster-Iskenius U 1985 Caudal dysplasia and femoral hypoplasia/unusual facies syndrome: different manifestations of the same disorder? European Journal of Paediatrics 144 (1): 80–82

Sadler T W 1980 Effects of maternal diabetes on early embryogenesis. II Hyperglycaemia induced exencephaly. Teratology 21: 349–356

Stubbs S M, Dodderidge M C, John P N, Steel J M, Wright A D 1987 Haemoglobin A_1 and congenital malformation. Diabetic Medicine 4: 156–159

Tallarigo L, Giampreto O, Penno G, Miccoli R, Gregori G, Navalesi R 1986 Relation of glucose tolerance to complications in pregnancy in non-diabetic women. New England Journal of Medicine 315 (16) 989–992

Watkins P J 1982 Congenital malformations and blood glucose control in diabetic pregnancy. British Medical Journal 284: 1357–1358

Ylinen K, Raivio K, Teramo K 1981 Haemoglobin A_{1c} predicts the perinatal outcome in insulin dependent diabetic pregnancies. British Journal of Obstetrics and Gynaecology 88: 961–967

13

Fetal macrosomia[*]

The infants of diabetic mothers are traditionally portrayed as being big. The large size is due to an increase in both weight and length (Cardell 1953a, Farquhar 1965). The increase in weight is due to an increase in size and weight of most organs, which show cellular hypertrophy and hyperplasia. Extramedullary haematopoesis contributes to the extra weight, especially of the liver. In addition, there is an increase in body fat. Adipose tissue is prominent in the subcutaneous tissues and contributes to the round face and neck and the large chest and abdomen. Skinfold thickness reflects the increased adiposity being greater in infants of diabetic mothers than normal (Whitelaw 1977). Oedema does not play a part in the macrosomia; the total body water of infants of diabetic mothers is, in fact, reduced (Osler & Pedersen 1966).

The role of fetal hyperinsulinaemia

Maternal and hence fetal hyperglycaemia leading to fetal hyperinsulinaemia is generally held to be responsible for fetal macrosomia. Fetal pancreatic β-cell hyperplasia in stillborn infants of diabetic mothers was described by Cardell (1953b) and the hyperinsulinaemia hypothesis postulated by Pedersen and Osler (1961). Fetal hyperinsulinaemia has been confirmed by the finding of raised C-peptide levels in the cord blood of infants of diabetic mothers. C-peptide is secreted by the pancreas in equimolar amounts to insulin and its measurement is not influenced by maternal insulin antibodies which cross the placenta and may,

[*] Fetal macrosomia in this context is confined to those babies whose birthweight exceeds the 95th centile.

therefore, interfere with direct measurement of fetal insulin levels (Sosenko et al 1979). However, Knip et al (1983) have measured free and total immunoreactive insulin and C-peptide in cord blood at birth and found that the infants of diabetic mothers were markedly hyperinsulinaemic and that the hyper-insulinaemia was directly related to both macrosomia and neonatal hypoglycaemia. These authors found a discrepancy between the relative increase of free immunoreactive insulin and C-peptide and a low molar ratio of C-peptide to the insulin, suggesting either a decreased metabolic clearance of insulin or transplacental passage of insulin from maternal circulation in insulin-treated diabetics. The latter suggestion goes against the widely held belief that insulin does not cross the placental barrier, and more positive evidence is needed before this belief can be challenged. The tendency of the infants of diabetic mothers to become profoundly hypoglycaemic and the rapidity with which they dispose of a glucose load has been noted by many authors (Isles et al 1968, Sosenko et al 1982). Susa & Schwartz (1985) showed that chronic infusion of insulin into the fetus of the normal pregnant rhesus monkey caused fetal growth and hormone abnormalities similar to those found in human diabetic pregnancy; they concluded that hyperinsulinaemia was the cause of the fetal macrosomia.

The role of insulin and related peptides in fetal growth has been comprehensively examined by Milner & Hill (1984). The human β-cell is recognizable from the 10th week of gestation and insulin is found in fetal blood from about the 12th week onwards. Potter et al (1986) examined maternal plasma amino acid levels in early pregnancy and found that the post-prandial levels of some individual amino acids were elevated in diabetes. Since amino acids are important in early islet development and insulin se-cretion, the elevated post-prandial levels found in diabetics may contribute to fetal islet hypertrophy and hyperinsulinaemia. The secretion of insulin does not, however, become responsive to glucose until about 28 weeks. Before this, insulin secreted possibly under amino acid stimulation causes a wide variety of cells to synthesize and secrete growth stimulating peptides. Insulin growth factor I (IGFI) results from this mechanism, while Insulin growth factor II (IGFII) is produced by a different mech-anism in which the placenta or one of its hormones plays a part. Thus insulin has a dual role in fetal growth: in early pregnancy it brings about the growth and development of the cells, in late pregnancy, secreted in response to fetal blood glucose levels, it stimulates the laying down of fat. In diabetic pregnancy the fetal pancreas is being over-stimulated and an excessive amount of fat deposition results.

In the diabetic rat, Kim et al (1980) found there was an increase in cell proliferation rate, leading to macrosomia. These workers also found macrosomia was more likely to occur in mildly diabetic animals rather than in those more severely affected, perhaps because more severe disease reduces the transport of metabolites across the placenta to the fetus. In human diabetic pregnancy severe maternal diabetes complicated by vasculopathy may result in fetal intrauterine growth retardation by the same mechanism. Fetal hyperinsulinaemia leads to an increased deposition of glycogen in the liver and also stimulates triglyceride synthesis in adipose cells, causing these cells to hypertrophy thus leading to an increase in the quantity of subcutaneous fat (Pedersen 1977). Szabo & Szabo (1974) also emphasized the importance of triglyceride in the pathogenesis of fetal adiposity in infants of diabetic mothers. They hypothesize that the increased levels of free fatty acids found in diabetic mothers result in an accelerated transfer of these substances across the placenta to be taken up by fetal adipocytes and esterified to triglycerides. Knopp et al (1986) have recently shown that a transplacental free fatty acid gradient exists in the direction of the fetus and is proportional to the maternal free fatty acid concentration.

Many investigators have examined the relationship between the levels of maternal blood glucose and haemoglobin A_1 level with both the birthweight of the baby and its subcutaneous fat. In the non-diabetic, macrosomia is only related to maternal hyperglycaemia when the birthweight is above the 99th centile and the mean blood glucose above the 88th centile. So, clearly factors other than maternal hyperglycaemia play a part in the macrosomia (Oats et al 1980). This is borne out by the fact that, although the incidence of diabetes is increased among the mothers of macrosomic infants, only a small minority of all women giving birth to such babies show any abnormality of carbohydrate metabolism (Madanlon et al 1980).

Stevenson et al (1982) drew attention to the categories of primary and secondary growth excess of prenatal onset. Primary growth excess is related to a basic problem in the skeletal cells, leading to excessive growth. Secondary growth excess is the result of maternal factors operating during pregnancy and leading to excessive growth of basically normal cells. Maternal diabetes is the classic example of this latter condition. In addition to the primary and secondary growth categories, there are macrosomic babies who do not fall easily into either of these categories. They are often the offspring of obese women. Subcutaneous maternal fat in excess is not necessarily associated with greater than average birthweight but it usually is, and fat mothers tend to have big babies who are both macrosomic and have increased subcutaneous fat (Whitelaw 1976). Hyperinsulinaemia may occur in normoglycaemic babies and is also seen in erythroblastosis fetalis (Van Asshe et al 1970, Falorini et al 1972). Neither of these situations is associated with macrosomia. Burke et al (1979) described a twin pregnancy occurring in a well-controlled diabetic woman. Only one of the babies was macrosomic. In the experimental animal, Mintz & Chez (1976) showed that an intact neurohypophysis was necessary for hyperglycaemia to cause fetal hyperinsulinaemia. These observations do not invalidate the hypothesis that fetal hyperinsulinaemia is the cause of fetal macrosomia, but lend support to the view of Shelley et al (1975) that other hormones may also influence the levels of fetal glucose and insulin and hence the development of macrosomia. This may be the explanation for the occurrence of fetal macrosomia even when maternal diabetic control is such that the degree of both maternal and fetal hyperglycaemia is likely to be small (see below). If the fetus becomes hypoxic (see Ch. 11) and is also hyperglycaemic, there will be an increased metabolism of glucose through the hexose monophosphate shunt pathway, resulting in an exaggerated synthesis of triglycerides in fetal adipose tissue, so increasing fetal macrosomia (Macfarlane & Tsakalakos 1983).

Clinical aspects

The clinician is interested in fetal macrosomia both as an indicator of the effect which the maternal diabetes is having on the fetus and because of the difficulties it is likely to cause with delivery. The generally held view that badly controlled diabetics are more likely to have macrosomic babies has come under very careful scrutiny, since it infers that by controlling maternal blood glucose levels closely macrosomia can be avoided. No consistent relationship has been found between maternal blood glucose levels or haemoglobin A_1 levels during pregnancy and birthweight. A relationship has, however, been found between maternal blood glucose levels in the last trimester of pregnancy and skinfold thickness (Whitelaw 1977). Stubbs et al (1981) found a similar correlation in diabetic pregnancy and also a relationship between skinfold thickness and third trimester haemoglobin A_1 levels. Williams et al (1986), in a series of 95 diabetic women who had macrosomic babies, found that the risk of macrosomia was doubled in women with mean glucose concentrations equal to or greater than 7.2 mmol/ℓ, was increased one-and-a-half times in women with insulin dosages more than 80 units/day and was trebled in women whose weight exceeded 80 kg. These findings emphasized the important clinical point that several maternal factors in addition to hyperglycaemia play a part in the development of macrosomia in the infants of diabetic women. Any lack of correlation between diabetic control and birthweight is somewhat academic in clinical practice, since if bad control gives rise to fatter babies they are likely to be big and, therefore, difficult to deliver. The important point that must be made is that, although immaculate control of maternal diabetes may lower the overall incidence of macrosomia, it may also be associated in an individual case with a macrosomic baby. Knight et al (1983) described the case of a woman whose diabetes was strictly controlled by continuous subcutaneous infusion of insulin from before conception to the time of delivery. The baby weighed 4.9 kg and had a typical diabetic appearance. Viser et al (1984) reported that continuous subcutaneous insulin infusions decreased the incidence of macrosomia but that, nevertheless, macrosomia was still common even though maternal mean blood glucose and haemoglobin A_1 levels were generally very good with this regimen.

The incidence of macrosomia at King's College Hospital in 100 well-controlled diabetic women was 30% (Brudenell & Carr 1984). In that series macrosomia was not affected by maternal age, parity, height, duration of diabetes, insulin requirement, blood glucose or haemoglobin A_1 levels. Vascular complications and smoking made the development of macrosomia less likely. The only significant factor which affected the development of macrosomia was gestational age at delivery. Allowing well-controlled women to go to full term gave a higher incidence of macrosomia than the previous policy of induction of labour and delivery between 37 and 38 weeks.

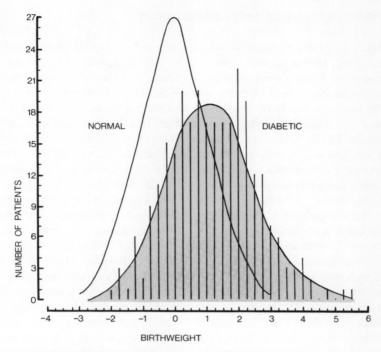

Fig. 13.1 Birthweight distribution of infants of diabetic mothers

The concept of macrosomic versus non-macrosomic babies in diabetic pregnancy has been examined by Bradley et al (1988). They examined the delivery details of 280 infants of diabetic mothers to see if there was a bimodal distribution in birthweights. In fact, the distribution of birthweight formed a unimodal normal distribution (Fig. 13.1). Furthermore, this distribution was shifted significantly to the right with a mean of 1.23 standard deviations, approximately 500 g. This accords with the fact that diabetic control is neither 'good' nor 'bad' but forms a continuous spectrum. Every diabetic woman will have a mean blood glucose greater than normal, so it is probable that every diabetic baby exceeds its genetic potential for growth (i.e is 'macrosomic') because of this, even though its actual birthweight may fall within the normal range. From the clinical point of view, however, the division into macrosomic and non-macrosomic is convenient and is certainly of help in managing late pregnancy and delivery (see Ch. 9).

Management of fetal macrosomia

Developing fetal macrosomia is detected by serial ultrasound scanning and is usually obvious by 30–32 weeks (Fig. 13.2). However, Flynn et al (1986) have recently studied 71 pregnancies in insulin-dependent diabetic women at King's College Hospital. The mean velocity of growth of the fetal abdominal circumference was calculated over a period from the first ultrasound scan, usually 12–16 weeks, to 24 weeks. The mean velocity of growth in macrosomic babies was significantly greater than in babies with normal birthweights, indicating that fetal growth is increased earlier than has been previously believed. The earlier that developing macrosomia can be detected the better, since it gives the diabetic physician a chance to check that maternal blood levels are being satisfactorily controlled. In a previous study to the one above, Fenech et al (1985), using serial fetal abdominal circumference measurements in 50 consecutive diabetic pregnancies, plotted probability graphs from 28 to 36 weeks. Two are illustrated (Fig. 13.3). If, for example, the abdominal circumference at 30 weeks is 25 cm, the probability of the predicted birthweight being less than the 75th centile is 40%; between the 75th and 95th centiles, also 40% but only a 20% chance that it will be greater than the 95th centile. If by 34 weeks the abdominal circumference is 29 cm, there is a 70% chance the baby will be macrosomic at birth, i.e. over the 95th centile. If this is the case then nothing further can be done and the problem is then for the obstetrician to decide when and how to deliver the baby. Bearing in mind that developing macrosomia is an indicator of the effect which the maternal diabetes, albeit well controlled, is having on the fetus, delivery earlier than full term will generally be advisable. The situation should usually be assessed at about 38 weeks: if, by this time, the baby is clearly macrosomic delivery should be expedited. Careful clinical assessment of maternal pelvis, extent of descent of the fetal head and cervical dilatation, together with a consideration of any past obstetric history, will generally indicate whether or not induction of labour is likely to lead to a successful vaginal delivery. If it is not, then delivery should be by planned caesarean section. Borderline cases can be allowed a short trial of labour. Delivery of the diabetic baby is not a time for heroic obstetrics. The risk of birth trauma is high when the baby is big in relation to the maternal pelvis, intracranial haemorrhage, shoulder dystocia and limb fractures being

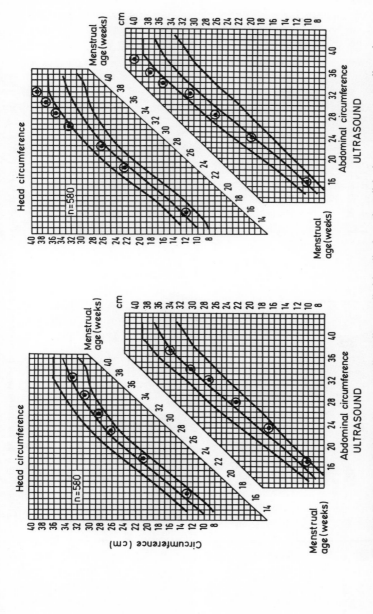

Fig. 13.2 Fetal growth charts in two equally well-controlled insulin-dependent diabetics: one grew normally and went into spontaneous labour at 39 weeks (BW 3.3 kg); the other was induced at 38 weeks (BW 4.3 kg). Both had spontaneous vaginal deliveries.

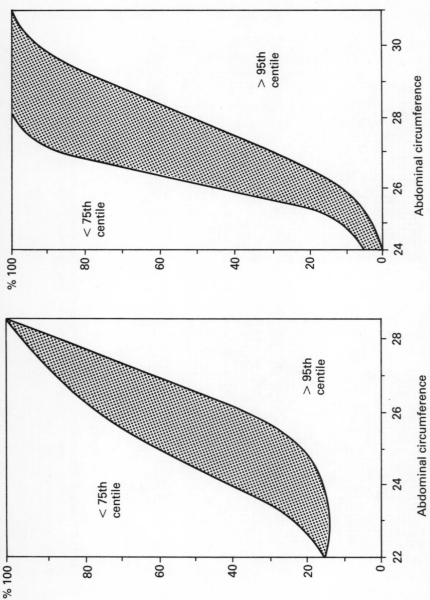

Fig. 13.3 Probability table for macrosomia in infants of diabetic mothers at 30th week (left) and 34th week (right)

the main hazards (Spellacy et al 1985). When these complications occur, the obstetric management can be judged to have been faulty since they would have been avoided by planned caesarean section. In passing, however, it should be pointed out that delivering a macrosomic baby by the abdominal route is not without its hazards and should only be performed by skilled obstetric surgeons. Difficulty in delivering the fetal head through the lower uterine segment incision may lead to extension of the incision laterally, with consequent risk of a broad ligament haematoma or ureteric damage. The risk to the baby is, of course, much less than with a difficult vaginal delivery and for this reason caesarean section is justified.

In future, careful clinical and ultrasound examination of the growing fetus, coupled with the known factors that predispose to macrosomia, *may* make some degree of control over excessive growth possible (e.g. by ensuring that maternal glucose control is really very tight and by encouraging obese women to lose weight before they become pregnant). The increasing risk of macrosomia when pregnancy is allowed to go to full term must be borne in mind and elective caesarean section carried out whenever vaginal delivery seems likely to be traumatic.

REFERENCES

Bradley 1988 British Medical Journal (in press)
Brudenell M, Carr J 1984 Conservative management of pregnancy in diabetic women. British Medical Journal 288: 1995
Burke B J, Savage D E, Sherriff R J, Dercor H G 1979 Diabetic twin pregnancy, an unequal result. Lancet i: 1372–1373
Cardell B S 1953a The infants of diabetic mothers. A morphological study. Journal of Obstetrics and Gynaecology of the British Empire 60: 834–853
Cardell B S 1953b Hypertrophy and hyperplasia of the pancreatic islets in newborn infants. Journal of Pathology and Bacteriology 66 (2): 335–346
Falorini A, Fracassini F, Massi-Benedette F, Amici A 1972 Glucose metabolism; plasma insulin and growth hormone secretion in newborn infants with erythroblastosis fetalis compared with normal newborn and those born to diabetic mothers. Pediatrics 49: 682–693
Farquhar J W 1965 The influence of maternal diabetes on fetus and child. In: Gardener D (ed) Recent advances in paediatrics. J and A Churchill, London, pp 121–153
Fenech F, Doddridge M, Pyke D A 1985 Fetal growth pattern in diabetic macrosomia. Presented to European Diabetic Pregnancy Study Group
Flynn M D, Doddridge M, Watkins P, Brudenell M 1986 Presentation to the British Diabetic Association
Isles T E, Dickson M, Farquhar J M 1968 Glucose Tolerance and plasma insulin in newborn infants of diabetic mothers. Pediatrics Research 2: 198–208

Kim Y S, Jatoi I, Kim Y 1980 Neonatal macrosomia in maternal diabetes. Diabetologia 18: 407–411

Knopp R H, Warth M R, Charles D et al 1986 Lipoprotein metabolism in pregnancy, fat transport to the fetus and the effects of diabetes. Biology of the Neonate 50: 297–317

Knight G, Worth R C, Ward J D 1983 Macrosomy despite a well controlled diabetic pregnancy. Lancet iv: 1431

Knip M, Lantala P, Leppaluoto J, Akerblom H K, Konvalainen K 1983 Relation of enteroinsular hormones at birth to macrosomia and neonatal hypoglycaemia in infants of diabetic mothers. Journal of Pediatrics 103(4): 603–611

Madanlon H D, Dorchester W L, Thorosian A, Freeman R K 1980 Macrosomia—maternal, fetal and neonatal implications. Obstetrics and Gynecology 55: 420

Macfarlane C M, Tsakalakos N 1983 Relative fetal hypoxia as a contributing factor to fetal macrosomia in diabetic pregnancy. Medical Hypothesis 11: 365–374

Milner R D G, Hill D J 1984 Fetal growth: the role of insulin and related peptides. Clinical Endocrinology 21: 415–433

Mintz D H, Chez R A 1976 Effects of diabetes mellitus on fetal growth and development. In: Fajan S S (ed) Diabetes mellitus. DHEW publication (NIH) 76–854, pp 256–264

Oats J N, Abell D A, Beisher H A, Broomhall G R 1980 Maternal glucose tolerance during pregnancy with excessive size infants. Obstetrics and Gynecology 55: 184–186

Osler M, Pedersen J 1960 The body composition of newborn infants of diabetic mothers. Pediatrics 26: 985–992

Pedersen J 1977 The pregnant diabetic and her newborn. 2nd Edition, Wilkins & Wilkins, Baltimore, p 129

Pedersen J, Osler M 1961 Hyperglycaemia as a cause of characteristic features of the foetus and newborn of diabetic mothers. Danish Medical Bulletin 8: 78–83

Potter J M, Green A, Cullen D R, Milner R D 1986 Amino acid profiles in early diabetic and non diabetic pregnancy. Diabetes Research and Clinical Practice 2 (3): 123–126

Shelley H J, Basset J M, Milner R D G 1975 Control of carbohydrate metabolism in the fetus and newborn. British Medical Bulletin 31: 37–43

Sosenko I R, Kitzmuller J L, Loo S W, Blise P, Rubenstein A H, Gabbay K H 1979 Correlation of increased cord C-peptide levels with macrosomia and hypoglycaemia. New England Medical Journal 301: 859–862

Sosenko J M, Kitzmuller J L, Fluckiger R, Loo S W, Younger D M, Gabbay K H 1982 Umbilical cord glycosylated haemoglobin in infants of diabetic mothers: relationship to neonatal hypoglycaemia, macrosomia and serum cord C-peptide. Diabetes Care 5(6): 566–570

Spellacy W N, Miller S, Windegar A, Pelerson P Q 1985 Macrosomia; maternal characteristics and infant complications. Obstetrics and Gynecology 66(2): 158–161

Stevenson D K, Hopper A O, Cohen R S, Bucalo L R, Kerner J A, Sunshine P 1982 Macrosomia; causes and consequences. Journal of Pediatrics 150(4): 515–520

Stubbs S M, Leslie R D J, John P N 1981 Fetal macrosomy and maternal diabetic control in pregnancy. British Medical Journal 282: 439–440

Susa J B, Schwartz R 1985 Effects of hyperinsulinaemia in the primate fetus. Diabetes 34, Suppl 2: 36–41

Szabo A J, Szabo O 1974 Placental free fatty-acid transfer and fetal adipose tissue development. An explanation of fetal adiposity in infants of diabetic mothers. Lancet ii: 498–499

Van Asshe F A, Fepts W, de Gasparo M, Renaer M 1970 The endocrine pancreas in erythroblastosis fetalis. Biology of the Neonate 15: 176–185

Viser G H A, Van Ballagooie E, Slunter W J 1984 Blood Glucose control in pregnancy using continuous subcutaneous insulin infusions. Lancet i: 284–285

Whitelaw A G L 1976 Influence of maternal obesity on subcutaneous fat in the newborn. British Medical Journal 1: 985–986

Whitelaw A G L 1977 Subcutaneous fat in newborn infants of diabetic mothers: an indication of quality of diabetic control. Lancet i: 15–18

Williams S P, Leveno K J, Guzick D S, Williams M L, Whalley P J 1986 Glucose threshold for macrosomia in pregnancy complicated by diabetes. American Journal of Obstetrics and Gynecology 154: 470–475

14

The placenta

The diabetic placenta has been the subject of many morphological studies but no consistent pattern of change from normal has emerged. This may be in part because of the many variables which exist in diabetic states in pregnancy, ranging from gestational diabetes through to established diabetes with vasculopathy. The effect of superimposed disease, especially hypertension and pre-eclampsia, which themselves produce changes in the placenta, makes the picture even more confusing. A variant of considerable importance is the maturity of the placenta examined, since changes that may be apparent in the last 1 or 2 weeks of pregnancy may be absent at an earlier stage. The effect which control of maternal diabetes has on placental morphology is uncertain, but in so far as control affects the fetus it is also likely to affect the placenta; indeed, the placental changes may precede or be, in part, responsible for the changes in the fetus.

Gross appearance

The placentae of diabetic women are usually heavier than normal (Nummi 1972), depending on the weight of the fetus they serve: macrosomic babies have large placentae. The placenta appears bulky and oedematous; the umbilical cord in particular is often swollen and oedematous, sometimes making ligation difficult. The incidence of a single umbilical artery is increased, being 3–5% in diabetics as opposed to 1% in the general population. This is probably the result of the general tendency toward increased congenital abnormality. Infarcts are not increased in size or number, although controversy still exists on this point (Naeye 1978).

Microscopic appearances
Light microscopy

Although not pathognomic for maternal diabetes, about 60% of diabetic placentas have villi which are either immature or show accelerated maturation. The remaining 40% have villi which show a normal degree of morphological maturity. Villus oedema is common and villus vascularity varies as with villus length between the hypovascular, normal, and prominent and congested. Often there is an excess of villi which have undergone fibrinoid necrosis. Although proliferative endarteritis is often found in the fetal stem arteries, the changes do not resemble those seen in diabetic angiopathy (Fox 1978). The trophoblast envelope of the villi is often broad, with large and active cells in the cytotrophoblast and a prominent syncytiotrophoblastic layer, resulting in the formation of many syncytial sprouts. These changes often result in narrowing of the intervillus space which becomes slitlike (Naeye 1981).

Electron microscopy

A detailed description of the findings of electron microscopical studies of the diabetic placenta has been given by Fox (1978) and Naeye (1978). Once again, there is no specific constant or uniform pattern, although the occurrence of a prominent villus cytotrophoblastic layer is confirmed. Focal necrosis of areas of syncytiotrophoblast are seen and there is also often thickening of the trophoblastic basement membrane. One observation may be significant: in normal human placentae the brush border membranes of the syncytiotrophoblast are rich in insulin receptors (Whitsett 1980); however, the binding of insulin by specific receptors is decreased in the placentae of diabetics (Harrison et al 1977), so that it would be expected that there would be a morphological change to identify the functionally altered brush border. Teasdale & Jean Jaques (1986), investigating the morphology of the placental micro villous membrane in human diabetic placentae, found a significant increase in the surface density of microvilli compared with normal placentae. They conclude that the already large villous surface area in the diabetic placenta can be significantly enlarged by the microvilli, thus increasing its functional capacity.

Utero-placental circulation

The morphology of the utero-placental vasculature has been examined by a number of investigators using placental bed biopsies obtained at caesarean section. Pinkerton (1963) did not find any abnormality, but Driscoll (1965) found arteriolar medial hypertrophy and/or hyalinization with narrowing of the lumen in the decidual arteries. These changes are, however, also found in hypertensive pregnancy and are thus not truly characteristic of diabetes alone. There is therefore no firm evidence of damage to the vessels supplying blood to the maternal side of the placenta in diabetic pregnancy uncomplicated by hypertension.

Conclusions

The lack of a uniform abnormality in the diabetic placenta is not surprising, given the complexity of diabetes itself and the effects of other superimposed factors. In general, the degree of placental abnormality is most marked in severe and badly controlled diabetics, but identical changes may be found in the placenta in gestational diabetic pregnancy. There is no obvious reason to suppose that the diabetic placenta is functionally impaired: the often large size of the infant is an indication of good placental transfer of nutrients. The large size of the placenta resulting from cellular hyperplasia suggests not only an increased transfer capability but also an increased synthetic function. Neither is hyperglycaemia itself the sole factor behind placental abnormality, since a large placenta may occur in well-controlled diabetic pregnancy. It is likely, however, that in some pregnancies placental failure to transfer oxygen develops in late pregnancy and is responsible for the classic late intrauterine death of the fetus. The narrowing of the intervillous space which follows the trophoblast changes noted above might bring this about. This possibility awaits further investigation. There is at present no direct evidence, but the results of fetal blood sampling in utero in late pregnancy (cordocentesis) suggest that hypoxia is not uncommon in late diabetic pregnancy and may on occasion be fatal (see Ch. 11).

REFERENCES

Driscoll S G 1965 The pathology of pregnancy complicated by diabetes
  mellitus. Medical Clinics of North America 49: 1053–1067
Fox H 1978 Placenta in maternal disorders. In: Fox H, Elston C W (eds)
  Pathology of the placenta. W B Saunders, London, pp 224–230
Harrison L C, Billington T, Clark S, Nichols R, East I, Martin F I R 1977
  Decreased binding of insulin receptors on placental membranes from diabetic
  mothers. Journal of Clinical Endocrinology and Metabolism 44: 206–209
Naeye R L 1978 The outcome of diabetic pregnancies: a prospective study. In:
  Pregnancy, metabolism, diabetes and the fetus. Ciba Foundation Symposium
  No 63, pp 227–241
Naeye R L 1981 In: Naeye R L (ed) Perinatal diseases. Williams and Wilkins,
  London, pp 244–285
Nummi S 1972 Relative weight of the placenta and perinatal mortality. Acta
  Obstetrica et Gynecologica Scandinavia. Suppl 17: 1–69
Pinkerton J H M 1963 The placental bed arterioles in diabetes. Proceedings of
  the Royal Society of Medicine 56: 1021–1022
Teasdale F, Jean Jaques G 1986 Placenta 7 (1): 81–88
Whitsett J A 1980 Specialisations in plasma membranes of the human placenta.
  Journal of Pediatrics 96: 600–604

15

The infant of the diabetic mother (IDM)

The best descripton of an infant who has been affected by maternal diabetes has been given by Farquhar (1959):

> The infants are remarkable not only because like fetal versions of Shadrach, Meshach and Abednego they emerge at least alive from within the firey furnace of diabetes mellitus but because they resemble one another so closely that they might be related. They are plump, sleek, liberally coated with vernix caseosa, full faced and plethoric. The umbilical cord and the placenta share in the gigantism. During their first 24 or more hours of extrauterine life they lie on their backs bloated and flushed, their legs flexed and abducted, their lightly closed hands on each side of the head, the abdomen prominent and the respiration sighing. They convey a distinct impression of having had such a surfeit of food and fluid pressed upon them by an insistent hostess that they desire only peace so that they might recover from their excesses and on the second day their resentment of the slightest noise improves the analogy while their trembling anxiety seems to speak of intrauterine indiscretions of which we know nothing.

The head may appear disproportionately small but, in fact, the mean head circumference after 37 weeks is greater than average (Gamsu 1978). The infants are often hirsute. The respiratory rate tends to be rapid (transient tachypnoea of the newborn) and this has sometimes been a source of confusion with the true respiratory distress syndrome. The characteristic features of IDM disappear in the first 2 weeks, and thereafter each baby develops its own individual characteristic. Not all infants of diabetic mothers present the classic picture, indeed many appear to be completely normal. Whilst it is accepted that poor maternal diabetic control is associated with a greater incidence of macrosomia, the characteristic 'tomato baby' appearance may also be the end product of a perfectly controlled diabetic pregnancy. The management of all infants of diabetic mothers, whether presenting the characteristic appearance or not, calls for expert paediatric care and is best left in the hands of neonatal paediatricians who are familiar with the particular problems.

Neonatal morbidity

Neonatal morbidity in these infants has changed considerably over the past 20 years and many of them have an apparently normal, uncomplicated passage through the first weeks of life. Formerly at King's College Hospital it was routine for an IDM to be taken immediately after birth to the special care baby unit, but nowadays the majority, after any necessary initial resuscitation, accompany the mother to the lying-in ward in the normal way.

Asphyxia

Asphyxia is more common in the IDM (Gamsu 1978), reflecting in part the increased incidence of fetal distress in labour (Brudenell 1978). Hypoxaemia and hyperinsulinaemia are inversely correlated in the cord blood, indicating that those babies most affected in utero by maternal hyperglycaemia are the ones most likely to be hypoxic (MacFarlane & Tsakalakos 1985). About one-third of all cases will require intubation, but this figure includes a number of preterm and other compromised infants so that the majority do not now require intubation. Metabolic acidosis (pH < 7.25) is seen in about 10% and may require intravenous sodium bicarbonate if it persists or worsens.

Respiratory distress syndrome (RDS) (See also Ch. 8)

The importance of RDS as a cause of perinatal mortality has diminished sharply in recent times, although it remains a potential hazard for the preterm IDM. Routine amniocentesis before delivery to measure the fetal lung maturity by means of lecithin/sphyngomyelin ratio estimations or the presence of phosphatidyl glycerol has been abandoned, except where delivery seems likely to take place before the 32nd week. In this very preterm situation an indication of lung maturity allows consideration to be given to its acceleration by means of administered corticosteroids (Liggins & Howie 1972). The management of RDS calls for expert neonatal paediatric care. The diagnosis is confirmed by the typical 'air bronchogram' appearance of the chest X-ray. Rigorous prevention of hypothermia, prompt raising of the ambient O_2 concentration and, if necessary, intermittent positive pressure ventilation are given to maintain an aortic oxygen tension of 70–99 mmHg (9.3–12.0 kPa). Only very premature infants are likely to succumb to this cause, given good modern neonatal paediatric care.

Hypoglycaemia

Blood glucose levels of 1.1 mmol/l occur more frequently in the IDM than in infants of non-diabetic mothers of equal maturity. The lowest blood glucose levels are seen in the first hour of life, after which the concentration begins to rise. Andersen et al (1985) demonstrated the influence of maternal plasma glucose concentration at delivery on the risk of neonatal hypoglycaemia. The higher the maternal glucose level the higher the cord plasma glucose level and the greater the risk of neonatal hypoglycaemia 2 hours after delivery. No IDM became hypoglycaemic when the maternal glucose level was less than 7.1 mmol/l. Hypoglycaemia is more common in macrosomic babies or after birth asphyxia. It is usually asymptomatic but apnoeic attacks, hypotonia, hypothermia, extreme excitability and tremulousness, rolling eye movements and frank convulsions are suggestive of the condition (Gamsu 1978). Hypoglycaemia results from hyperinsulinaemia (Cornblath & Schwartz 1976), which in turn is a reflection of maternal hyperglycaemia. A number of writers have found a correlation between maternal blood glucose levels in late pregnancy and neonatal hypoglycaemia (Pedersen 1967), Gillmer et al 1975, Haworth & Dilling 1976). Beard et al (1971) found an increased rate of disposal of a glucose load in the IDM by comparison with non-diabetics. Whether hyperinsulinaemia is the sole cause of neonatal hypoglycaemia is debatable. Not all studies have found a correlation between the condition and the level of insulin in the cord blood or maternal levels of glucose in late pregnancy (Martin et al 1975). These authors suggested that there is a failure to maintain basal glucose homeostasis after birth. This could be due to excessive uptake of glucose by the tissues from the circulation and/or a suppressed production of glucose from the liver. The part played by glucagon was examined by Bloom & Johnson (1972); they found an impaired glucagon increase in the IDM after birth and thought it a significant feature in their hypoglycaemia. As with macrosomia, neonatal hypoglycaemia may occur in very well-controlled diabetics so it is entirely possible that the simple and attractive hyperinsulinaemia theory may not be the whole explanation for either macrosomia or neonatal hypoglycaemia. Whatever its causation, prolonged hypoglycaemia in these infants is to be avoided for fear of long-term neurological sequelae: these are unlikely in the asymptomatic case (Haworth et al 1976) but prolonged hypoglycaemia with symptoms does carry the risk of irreversible neurological damage (Gamsu 1978). Breastfeeding is commenced shortly after birth and capillary blood glucose measured at 2 hours and 4 hours. If the level is less than 2.5 mmol/l on both occasions and the level is confirmed on a venous sample intravenous glucose is commenced and continued until a sustained rise in glucose levels greater than 2.5 mmol/l is obtained. When maternal non-insulin-dependent diabetes is being treated with sulfonylurea drugs (e.g. chlorpropamide, glibenclamide), these should be discontinued at least 2 days before delivery is anticipated, since they cross the placenta and may cause intractable neonatal hypoglycaemia (Kemball et al 1970). Exchange transfusion may have to be performed in these cases.

Hypocalcaemia and hypomagnesaemia

Neonatal hypocalcaemia (serum calcium < 1.65 mmol/l) and hypomagnesaemia (serum magnesium < 0.62 mmol/l) occur more frequently in the IDM. Tsang et al (1972) confirmed the findings of the earlier writers. The cause is not certain and the condition is relatively uncommon. Mimouni et al (1986) examined the possibility that polycythaemia might be a causal factor. They found no correlation between the haematocrit in the IDM and serum calcium or magnesium. A significant correlation did exist, however, between hypocalcaemia and hypomagnesaemia. The symptoms of hypocalcaemia occur in the first 48 hours of life—neuromuscular excitability, apnoeic spells and fits. Blood should be taken for calcium and magnesium estimations. If the levels are low, a slow intravenous infusion of calcium gluconate 5% or 10% (50–100 mg/kg) and, when necessary, intramuscular magnesium sulphate 50% (0.1 ml/kg) are given.

Polycythaemia

Although neonatal haematocrit is influenced by the timing of cord clamping and the extent of placental transfusion at birth, the IDM usually has a higher haematocrit than normal. Even with early clamping of the cord the mean haematocrit in a series of infants born at King's College Hospital was 64.2% at 2–4 hours, rising to 67.3% at 4–8 hours. Thirty-four per cent of these IDMs had a haematocrit of 70% or more during the first 8 hours after birth (Gamsu 1978). Venesection is recommended if the 2-hour figure is more than 70% (21 g% of Hb); 10–15% of the infant's blood volume is removed in aliquots of 5–10 ml and replaced with albumen or plasma in what amounts to a partial exchange transfusion. High levels of haematocrit may require as much as 20% of the infant's blood volume to be treated in this way if the hyperviscosity associated with polycythaemia (Kontrass 1972) is to be avoided. Shannon et al (1976) measured the cord blood erythropoetin in infants of well-managed diabetic mothers and found that it was no higher than normal. It was highest in infants after vaginal delivery and was inversely related to umbilical cord pH. Cord blood erythropoetin levels are strongly influenced by perinatal events, but the response of the IDM was normal, suggesting that polycythaemia is an adaptive process and not a primary abnormality of erythropoesis. It is characteristically a response to intrauterine fetal anoxia. The increased maternal levels of HbA_1 in the maternal circulation might cause a degree of fetal anoxia, since HbA_1 has a decreased reactivity to 2,3-diphosphoglycerate and increased affinity for oxygen. It would therefore transfer oxygen less readily across the placenta. This is not the sole explanation for intrauterine fetal anoxia but it is a contributory factor (see Ch. 11). In the last 5 years at King's, polycythaemia has become less of a problem than previously and venesection is now only rarely needed.

Jaundice

Hyperbilirubinaemia may result from neonatal polycythaemia. It occurred in 30% of the infants in an earlier King's series (Gamsu 1978) but it is much less common nowadays. Other contributors to hyperbilirubinaemia are bruising, including cephalhaematoma, following a traumatic delivery, blood group incompatibility and sepsis. Jaundice is more likely to occur in premature babies and in those who have had respiratory distress. Venesection of poly-cythaemic babies does not reduce the incidence of jaundice, although it may reduce its severity. A careful check on the level of bilirubin in the IDM is clearly necessary and phototherapy or rarely exchange transfusion is carried out as required.

Thrombosis

Renal vein thrombosis was reported as a complication in the IDM by Takeuchi & Benirscke (1961), and there have been sporadic reports since then. Samarrai et al (1984) described a case discovered at the post mortem examination of a stillborn IDM: there was extensive thrombosis from main to cortical branches of one renal vein, causing infarction of the kidney. Similar less severe changes were found in the other kidney. This complication has not been observed at King's in the last 20 years and is probably very rare in modern clinical practice. This in turn reflects a diminished incidence of polycythaemia, or its prompt treatment when it occurs, since this condition is the likely ante-cedent to such thromboses.

Birth trauma

Birth trauma is the result of difficult vaginal delivery, more common in diabetic labour, complicated by fetal macrosomia. Difficult vaginal delivery has no place in the modern management of diabetic pregnancy. Macrosomia should be recognized by ante-natal ultrasound scanning and, if there is any prospect of dispro-portion, the baby delivered by planned caesarean section. Borderline cases are many, however, and fine obstetric judge-ment is called for (see Ch. 9).

Morphology

Systematic study of the organs and tissues of IDMs has been restricted in recent years because of the falling perinatal mortality rate. The early reports and later work have been well reviewed by Haust (1981). The changes the various observers report are necessarily related to perinatal deaths and represent extremes of changes in infants seriously affected by maternal diabetes. In modern practice such perinatal deaths should be rare so the importance of these changes to the clinician is less than it was previously.

Long-term outlook for IDMs

The infants of diabetic mothers have a greater than average chance of developing diabetes in later life but the actual risk is of the order of 1% as against 0.1% in infants of mothers who are not diabetic. (Breidahl 1966, White 1960). This is an acceptable risk but the individuals concerned should be made aware of it especially the women when they become pregnant. Macrosomic babies tend to become obese and obesity may then be associated with abnormal glucose tolerance (Farquhar 1969, Vohr et al 1979). The IDM, macrosomic or otherwise, usually exhibits normal physical development, however (Stark & Farquhar 1975). Persson et al (1986) followed 53 children of insulin-dependent diabetic mothers and 20 children of gestational diabetic mothers. At 5 and 11 years the majority of the children were of normal height and weight. Mental development is also usually normal, although a slight increase in neurological deficit and low IQ has been reported (Cummins & Norish 1980). Whether this is due to neonatal hypoglycaemia is disputed. Gamsu (1978) reports that prolonged symptomatic hypoglycaemia does carry the risk of neurological damage, but Haworth et al (1976) could find no correlation between the two. Petersen et al (1988) relate early growth delay to developmental impairment at age 4 and recommend that any IDM who has shown impaired growth between 8 and 14 weeks should be specially screened in childhood. In commenting on this paper Harper & Morrow (1988) point out the difficulties in demonstrating true growth impairment in early pregnancy.

The overall prognosis for the IDM is good, but expert neonatal paediatric care is an essential part of their management.

REFERENCES

Andersen O, Hertel J, Schmolker L, Kuhl C (1985) Influence of maternal plasma glucose concentration on the risk of hypoglycaemia in infants of insulin dependent diabetic mothers. Acta Paediatrica Scandinavia 74 (2): 268–273

Beard R W, Turner R C, Oakley N 1971 Fetal response to glucose loading. Fetal blood glucose and insulin responses in normal and diabetic pregnancies. Postgraduate Medical Journal 47: 68–70

Bloom S R, Johnson D I 1972 Failure of glucose release in infants of diabetic mothers. British Medical Journal 4: 453

Breidahl H D 1966 The growth and development of children born to mothers with diabetes. Medical Journal of Austria 1: 268

Brudenell J M 1978 Delivering the infant of the diabetic mother. Journal of the Royal Society of Medicine 71: 207–211

Cornblath M, Schwartz R 1976 In: Shaffer A J, Markowitz N (eds) Major problems in clinical paediatrics vol 3, 2nd edition. Saunders, Philadelphia, p. 115

Cummins N, Norish M 1980 Follow up of children of diabetic mothers. Archives of Disease in Childhood 55: 259

Farquhar J W 1959 The child of the diabetic woman. Archives of Disease in Childhood 34: 76–96

Farquhar J W 1969 Prognosis for babies born to diabetic mothers in Edinburgh. Archives of Disease in Childhood 44: 36–40

Gamsu H R 1978 Neonatal morbidity in infants of diabetic mothers. Proceedings of the Royal Society of Medicine 71: 211–221

Gillmer M D G, Beard R W, Brooke F M, Oakley N W 1975 Part 1 Diurnal plasma glucose profile in normal and diabetic women. Part 2 Relation between maternal glucose tolerance and glucose metabolism in the newborn. British Medical Journal iii: 402–404

Harper M A, Morrow R J 1988 Early growth delay in diabetic pregnancy. British Medical Journal 296: 1005–1006

Haust M D 1981 In: Naeye R L, Kissane J M, Kasfria N (eds) Perinatal diseases. Williams and Wilkins, Baltimore/London, pp. 218–244

Haworth J C, McRae K N, Dilling L 1976 Prognosis of infants of diabetic mothers in relation to neonatal hypoglycaemia. Archives of Disease in Childhood 18: 471

Kemball M L, McIver C , Milner R D G, Nourse C H, Schiff D and Tiernan J R 1970 Neonatal hypoglycaemia in infants of diabetic mothers given sulphonylurea drugs in pregnancy. Archives of Disease in Childhood 45: 676–707

Kontrass S B 1972 Polycythaemia and hyperviscosity syndrome in infants and children. Pediatric Clinics of North America 19: 911–913

Liggins G C, Howie R N 1972 A controlled trial of antepartum glucocorticoid treatment for the prevention of the respiratory distress syndrome in premature infants. Pediatrics 50: 515–521

MacFarlane C M, Tsakalakos N 1985 Evidence of hyperinsulinaemia and hypoxaemia in the cord blood of neonates born to mothers with gestational diabetes. South African Medical Journal 67(3): 81–84

Martin F I, Dahlenberg G W, Russel J, Jeffrey P 1975 Neonatal hypoglycaemia in infants of insulin dependent diabetic mothers. Archives of Disease in Childhood. 50: 472–476

Mimouni F, Tsang R C, Hertzberg V S, Miodovnik M 1986 Polycythaemia, hypomagnesaemia and hypocalcaemia in infants of diabetic mothers. American Journal of Diseases of Childhood 140 (8): 798–800

Pedersen J 1967 The pregnant diabetic and her newborn. Munksgaard, Copenhagen, Williams and Wilkins, Baltimore

Persson B 1986 Long term morbidity in the offspring of diabetic mothers. Acta Endocrinologica. Supplement (Copenhagen) 277: 150–155

Petersen M B, Pedersen S A, Griesen G et al 1988 Early growth delay in diabetic pregnancy: relation to psychomotor development at age 4. British Medical Journal 296: 598–600

Samarrai S F, Kato A, Urano Y 1984 Renal vein thrombosis in stillborn infant of diabetic mother. Acta Pathologica Japan 34(6): 1441–1447

Shannon K, Davis J C, Kitzmuller J L, Fulcher S A, Kolnig H M 1986 Erythropoesis in infants of diabetic mothers. Pediatric Research 20 (2): 161–165

Stark M P K, Farquhar J W 1975 Children of diabetic mothers: subsequent weight. In: Camerini Davalos R A, Cole H S (eds) Early diabetes in early life. Academic Press, New York, p 587

Takeuchi A, Benirscke K 1961 Renal venous thrombosis of the newborn and its relation to maternal diabetes. Biologica Neonatorium 3: 237–256

Tsang R C, Kleinman L I, Sutherland J M, Light I G 1972 Hypocalcaemia in infants of diabetic mothers. Journal of Pediatrics 80: 384–395

Vohr B, Lipsitt L P, Oh W 1980 Somatic growth of children of diabetic mothers with reference to birth size. Journal of Paediatrics 92(2): 196–199

White P 1960 Childhood diabetes; its cause and influence on 2nd and 3rd generations. Diabetes 9: 345

16

Breastfeeding

Nearly 50% of mothers are reported to be breastfeeding 6 weeks after the birth of their babies in south east England (Martin & Monk 1982). Little information on lactation in diabetic mothers (Brudenell & Beard 1972) and its effects on insulin requirements has been available and this may, in part, be due to the fact that until recently diabetic babies were separated from their mothers at birth and taken to the special care baby unit. Nowadays the majority of IDMs do not require admission to this unit.

At King's College Hospital a survey was carried out in 1983 and it was found that 75% of the mothers were breastfeeding at 6 weeks (Whichelow & Doddridge 1983). Two important factors emerged. The first was that those babies who were encouraged to suckle within 12 hours of delivery were more likely to be weaned later than those put to the breast after that time. The second point concerns the advice given to increase the dietary allowance by 50 g carbohydrate as a contribution for the extra 600 calories needed in lactation. This increase is usually taken in the form of an extra pint of milk daily and two extra carbohydrate portions taken at tea and dinner or at dinner and the bedtime snack when the mother is more likely to be hungry rather than earlier in the day. Insulin requirements did not, on the whole, alter during lactation. This extra carbohydrate must be reduced when breastfeeding is stopped. Several mothers have anecdotally reported a decrease in their supply of milk if they have low blood sugars.

As has been mentioned, HbA_1 levels tend to go up after pregnancy when control is probably more relaxed. There was no significant difference in HbA_1 between those breastfeeding and those who chose to bottle feed. All diabetic mothers should be encouraged to breastfeed and this aim can usually be achieved by early suckling and an appropriate increase in maternal carbohydrate intake.

REFERENCES

Brudenell M, Beard R 1972 Diabetes in pregnancy. Clinics in Endocrinology and Metabolism 1: 673–695
Martin J, Monk J 1982 Infant feeding 1980. OPCS, London
Whichelow M J, Doddridge M C 1983 Lactation in diabetic women. British Medical Journal 287: 649–650

17

Family planning

For the average diabetic woman who wishes to have children a small family should be the aim. The problem of managing her diabetes and the possibility that long-term vascular complications will at some stage further impair her health make pregnancy and the addition of children into her life's equation much more of a burden than for the non-diabetic. The majority of IDD patients will be diagnosed before or during the time of their lives when they will wish to have children, so it is always appropriate to raise the question of family planning with them. Family planning for diabetic women should result in a planned family, not only in terms of numbers of children but also in the timing of conception, so as to ensure that it occurs at a time when diabetic control is optimal (see Ch. 4). The vascular complications of diabetes are more likely to arise after some years, so in general the diabetic woman should aim to have her children as early as possible in her reproductive life.

Traditional methods of contraception

Although the sheath and the contraceptive diaphragm have become somewhat unfashionable, they each offer the diabetic woman who is well motivated toward family planning and has a caring partner a reasonable degree of safety from unplanned pregnancy without risk of complications. The sheath used faithfully and combined with a contraceptive cream is slightly more reliable than the diaphragm used with a contraceptive cream or foam. Some couples will opt for one or other of these mechanical methods, and providing they have a clear understanding of the correct use of the devices can be encouraged to adopt this approach. The 'safe period' approach to contraception is generally regarded as unreliable when used on its own because ovulation by no means always occurs mid-cycle. It should not be recommended to diabetic women as a sole method of contraception, particularly as they often have irregular menstrual cycles. It does, nevertheless, provide an additional safety factor to the use of the sheath or cap or intrauterine device (IUD). For couples using these methods the avoidance of intercourse in mid-cycle will decrease the risk of failure.

The intrauterine device (IUD)

Next to the pill, the IUD offers a woman the best protection against an unplanned pregnancy. Although it has certain significant disadvantages, it has the important advantage that once placed in position the woman and her partner need take no further contraceptive measures. It is not a suitable method of contraception for nulliparous women unless no alternative method can be used. Of the disadvantages, the risk of intrauterine infections spreading to the tubes and causing salpingitis and possible tubal blockage is the most important. The risk of infection seems low in those women who have a regular and sole partner who is similarly faithful. It is likely that the overall risk of infection is greatest in those women who have several partners and are, therefore, at greater risk of infection with or without an IUD. The spread of infection is more rapid in diabetics, so diabetic women with an IUD should be advised to report at once any unusual lower abdominal pain or vaginal discharge. Several writers (Wiese 1974, Steel & Duncan 1980) reported a higher failure rate among diabetic IUD users than among non-diabetics, and it was suggested that this might be due, in the case of copper IUDs, to a lack of fibrinolytic activity in the endometrium (Larson 1977, Craig 1981) or to an increased deposition of sulphur on the device, copper or plastic, reflecting differences in endometrial metabolism in diabetics (Gosden et al 1982). A later paper by Wiese (1977) and a paper by Thiery (1982) failed to confirm a higher failure rate among diabetic IUD users. At King's College Hospital this method of contraception is offered to women on the same terms as non-diabetic women, but the use of the contraceptive foam or the avoidance of mid-cycle intercourse is recommended for the 1st year of use when the risk of failure is highest. Diabetic women using IUDs are likely to suffer from heavier or longer periods and from occasional extrusion of the device, as do non-diabetic women.

The contraceptive pill

The combined oral contraceptive pill is the most effective contraceptive method available to women at the present time. It does, however, carry a slight but definite risk of causing venous thrombo-embolism and it is this complication, rather than its minor effects on carbohydrate and lipid metabolism, which gives the greatest cause for concern in diabetic women. This is particularly the case among those diabetic women known to have vascular disease or hypertension. Against the risk of venous thrombo-embolism due to the pill must be set the risks of this condition in pregnancy, should the latter occur as the result of failure of other contraceptive methods. Diabetic women who wish to use the pill should be examined carefully for evidence of vasculopathy and hypertension. They should be encouraged to lose weight if they are obese and should be strongly discouraged from smoking. Adjustment of insulin dosage may be required but the majority of diabetic women suffer no disturbance of diabetic control when taking the pill. A recent study of 50 insulin-dependent diabetic women who took a non-alkylated oestrogen/progesterone compound for 1 year showed no significant increase in insulin requirement, urinary excretion of glucose, fasting glucose or haemoglobin A_{1c} levels. No pregnancies occurred and the continuation rate compared well with non-diabetic women on conventional combined oral contraception (Skouby et al 1985a). The most important advantage of the contraceptive pill is undoubtedly its acceptability to young sexually active women, for whom it provides a great feeling of security together with regular, mild, painless periods. Of the available formulations, the low dose triphasic pill containing varying amounts of ethinyloestradiol and levonorgestrel seems to have the smallest effect on carbohydrate and lipid metabolism and is the pill of first choice for diabetics (Skouby et al 1985b). True gestational diabetics—those who revert to the non-diabetic state after the pregnancy—do, nevertheless, often have some impairment of glucose tolerance so should probably avoid the combined pill. If, however, they do prefer this method, the low dose triphasic pill or progesterone only pill should be advised. Because of the risk of increasing vasculopathy with advancing age, the pill should not be prescribed for long periods in diabetic women and is not suitable for diabetic women over the age of 30.

The progesterone only pill

The progesterone only pill is not associated with an increased risk of venous thrombo-embolism and, from this point of view, is very suitable for the diabetic woman. However, it does sometimes cause irregular menstrual periods with intermenstrual spotting and it has a higher failure rate than the combined pill. The failure rate can be kept at acceptably low levels if the patient takes the pill without fail every day (Steel & Duncan 1981). The ideal time to try the progesterone only pill is after delivery, especially if the patient is breastfeeding. If it proves successful it can be continued thereafter. For the average non-pregnant diabetic woman who wishes to use oral contraception a low dose triphasic preparation with its regularity of menstrual periods and very low failure rate is probably the pill of choice but the progesterone only pill is a valuable alternative.

Laparoscopic sterilization

Laparoscopic sterilization is an easily performed gynaecological procedure with a very low failure rate (approximately 1 in 500 cases). It offers the diabetic woman who has completed her family the most satisfactory long-term solution to family planning problems. It should be freely available to diabetic women and should be offered to all pregnant diabetic women during the ante-natal period. Clearly it will be of no interest to those who wish to have more children, but by raising the subject with the patient at this time the doctor will be encouraging the woman to think about the importance of family limitation as well as family planning. It is normally performed 6 weeks post partum and the patient can usually be dealt with on a day case basis. Sterilization at the time of caesarean section is an option which should also be discussed with diabetic patients during the antenatal period.

In general, it will only be applicable to those women having planned repeat caesarean sections but, even in these cases, the obstetrician should generally reserve the right not to carry out the procedure at the time of the caesarean if the baby is, in any way, abnormal. Most patients are happy to agree to give the obstetrician this discretion so that if, for example, he sees the newborn baby developing respiratory difficulty he can postpone the sterilization until later. Vasectomy may be an appropriate alternative to female sterilization in some cases, but only if the male partner is certain that he will not want more children under any circumstances, bearing in mind that his diabetic wife's life expectancy may be reduced.

REFERENCES

Craig G M 1981 Diabetes, intra-uterine devices and fibrinolysis. British Medical Journal 283: 1184

Gosden C, Steel H, Ross A, Springbett A 1982 Intra-uterine contraceptive devices in diabetic women. Lancet i: 530–534

Larson B 1977 Fibrinolytic activity of the endometrium in diabetic women using copper IUCDs. Contraception 15: 711

Skouby S O, Jensen B M, Kuhl C et al 1985a Hormonal contraception in diabetic women. Acceptability and influence on diabetes control and ovarian function of a non-alkylated oestrogen/progesterone compound. Contraception 32: 23–31

Skouby S O, Kuhl C, Mølsted-Pederson L et al 1985b Triphasic oral contraception: metabolic effects in normal women and those with previous gestational diabetes. American Journal of Obstetrics and Gynecology 153: 528–533

Steel J, Duncan L J P 1980 Contraception for insulin dependent diabetics. Diabetes Care 3: 557–601

Steel J M, Duncan L J P 1981 The progesterone only pill in insulin dependent diabetics. British Journal of Family Planning 6: 108

Thiery M 1982 Intra-uterine contraceptive devices for diabetics. Lancet ii: 883

Wiese J 1974 Contraception in diabetic patients. Acta Endocrinologica Supplement (Copenhagen) 182: 87–94

Wiese J 1977 Intra-uterine contraception in diabetic women. Fertility and Sterility 28: 422–425

Addendum

Cordocentesis in diabetic pregnancy

Mention has already been made of cordocentesis (pp 61, 92) which is a technique for sampling fetal blood in utero. A 20 gauge needle is inserted under ultrasound control transabdominally into the umbilical cord at its placental insertion and a sample of fetal blood obtained. The sample may be arterial or venous, the distinction being made by an injection of a small quantity of saline at the end of the sample. The direction in which the saline flows identifies the vessel as an artery or vein. In a majority of cases the sample is found to have come from the umbilical vein. Cordocentesis is performed under local anaesthesia and has been shown by Daffos (1985) to be safe in skilled hands for both mother and fetus. It has been widely used for karyotyping blood cells in suspected haemoglobinopathy, in cases of rhesus isoimmunization and in the assessment of fetal well being in utero when the fetus is severely growth retarded (Nicolaides et al 1986).

At King's College Hospital cordocentesis has been employed by R J Bradley in different stages of diabetic pregnancy to study fetal oxygenation and glucose homeostasis. Fetal blood samples were obtained in 20 diabetic pregnancies at gestations ranging between 21 and 38 weeks and compared with the reference range established in normal pregnancy during fetal karyotyping. In the case of fetal oxygenation the results obtained indicate that PO_2 levels (Fig. 1) are significantly lower than normal and PCO_2 levels (Fig. 2) are significantly higher than normal in the cord blood of the diabetic fetus.

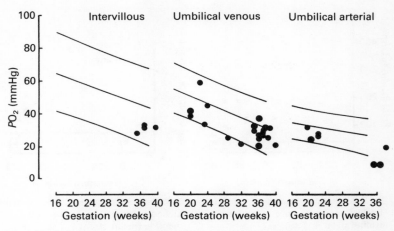

Fig. 1 Diabetic pregnancy. Fetal PO_2 (mean and 95% confidence intervals)

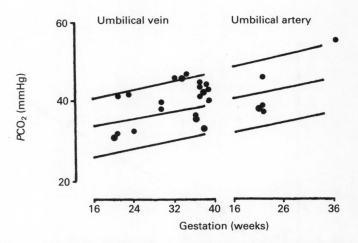

Fig. 2 Diabetic pregnancy. Fetal PCO_2 (mean and 95% confidence intervals)

Insulin and C-peptide levels were studied in 56 non-diabetic fetuses. There was no significant rise in levels of these two substances until the late stages of pregnancy. In 14 insulin diabetic pregnancies, however, fetal insulin and C-peptide levels were higher than normal in early pregnancy and rose to even higher levels as pregnancy advanced (Figs 3, 4).

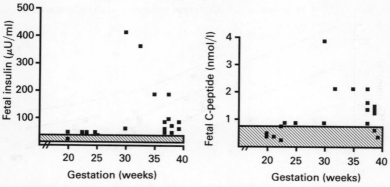

Fig. 3 Diabetic pregnancy. Fetal insulin. Hatched area, reference range for insulin (mean ± 2 SD)

Fig. 4 Diabetic pregnancy. Fetal C-peptide. Hatched area, reference range for C-peptide (mean ± 2 SD)

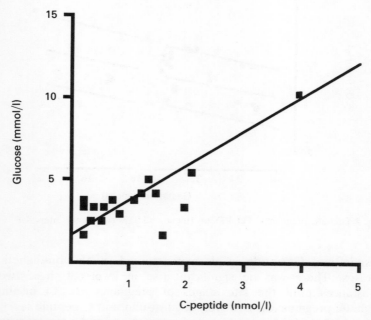

Fig. 5 Diabetic pregnancy. Correlation between fetal C-peptide and fetal glucose ($P < 0.001$, $r = 0.82$)

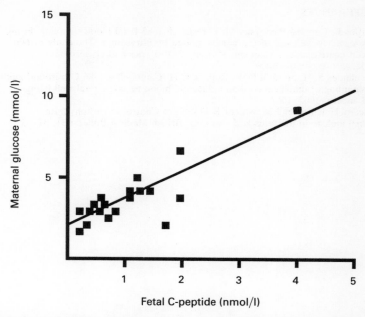

Fig. 6 Diabetic pregnancy. Correlation between fetal C-peptide and maternal glucose ($P < 0.001$, $r = 0.815$)

Fetal serum C-peptide levels were found to correlate with fetal glucose levels ($P < 0.001$). A correlation was also found between fetal C-peptide levels and maternal glucose levels at the time of sampling (Figs 5, 6), ($P < 0.002$) but not with mean glucose or haemoglobin A levels during pregnancy.

Surprisingly no correlation was found between fetal insulin levels and fetal macrosomia though there was a positive correlation between fetal insulin levels and the degree of fetal hypoxia. Fetal hyperinsulinaemia has been correlated with fetal macrosomia (see Ch. 13) and experimentally fetal consumption of oxygen is increased in the presence of hyperinsulinaemia (Shelley et al 1975). The number of diabetic pregnancies involved in this study so far is small and the patients are all well controlled but if the findings are confirmed in later studies new explanations may be needed for some of the phenomena of diabetic pregnancy. It seems likely that in the future cordocentesis may provide new insights into the problems of diabetic pregnancy.

REFERENCES

Daffos F, Capella–Pavlovsky M, Forestier F 1985 Fetal blood sampling during pregnancy with use of the needle guided by ultrasound. The study of 606 consecutive cases. American Journal of Obstetrics and Gynecology 153(6): 655–660

Nicolaides K H, Soothill P W, Rodeck C H, Campbell S 1986 Ultrasound-guided sampling of umbilical cord and placental blood to assess fetal well-being. Lancet i: 1065–1067

Shelley H J, Basset J M, Milner R D G 1975 Control of carbohydrate metabolism in the fetus and newborn. British Medical Bulletin 31: 37–43

Index

Index